Balance Your Brain, Balance Your Life

Balance Your Brain, Balance Your Life

28 Days to Feeling Better Than You Ever Have

Dr. Jay Lombard

and

Dr. Christian Renna

with Armin A. Brott

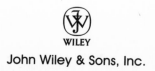

WILEY

John Wiley & Sons, Inc.

Published by John Wiley & Sons, Inc., Hoboken, New Jersey
Published simultaneously in Canada

Design and production by Navta Associates, Inc.

For general information about our other products and services, please contact our Customer Care Department within the United States at (800) 762-2974, outside the United States at (317) 572-3993 or fax (317) 572-4002.

Wiley also publishes its books in a variety of electronic formats. Some content that appears in print may not be available in electronic books. For more information about Wiley products, visit our web site at www.wiley.com.

Library of Congress Cataloging-in-Publication Data:

Lombard, Jay.
  Balance Your Brain, Balance Your Life: 28 Days to Feeling Better Than You
Ever Have /Jay Lombard and Christian Renna with Armin A. Brott.
      p. cm.
Includes bibliographical references and index.
  ISBN 0-471-37422-9 (cloth)
1. Health. 2. Mind and body. 3. Neurotransmitters. 4. Neurochemistry.
5. Homeostasis. I. Renna, Christian. II. Brott, Armin A. III. Title.
  RA776.5.L65 2003
  613—dc21
                                                              2003010757

Printed in the United States of America

10 9 8 7 6 5 4 3 2 1

To my daughter Julia Grace, my life's blessing.
—*from Jay*

To the many physicians and scientists who taught me the information I needed to know to contribute to this book. To Melinda, Gina, Nicki, and Maria for giving me the love, patience, and freedom necessary to complete the task. And to the countless numbers of patients who suffered my ignorance, endured my stubbornness, and taught me the greatest lessons of all by entrusting me with their health and diseases; it is to them I dedicate this book.
—*from Chris*

For Zoë, whose mind and body are growing at an incredible pace.
—*from Armin*

CONTENTS

ACKNOWLEDGMENTS

I'd like to thank James Levine, for his ability instantly to envision this project even in its most fledgling state and for nursing it to completion; Armin Brott for his uncanny ability to take complex material and make it accessible to people who have no background in neuroscience, which is quite a feat; Chris Renna, my coauthor and friend, for providing me the opportunity to experience his keen intellect and warm spirit; Carl Germano, for his insight on dietary suggestions and, more importantly, his great friendship; Tom Miller, without whose editorial direction this would have been an amorphous book about neurotransmitters without relevance to the reader; and to my wife, Rita, for her endless patience and endurance in living with an absent-minded, mad scientist/neurologist.

—*Jay Lombard*

Many thanks are due to Jay Lombard for his careful thinking and extensive knowledge of the workings of the human brain and the generous spirit with which he shared this information, and to Armin, Jim, and Tom for bringing it all together.

—*Christian Renna*

No matter how many names there on the cover, every book is a team effort. I'd like to thank the following people who helped make this project a reality. My parents, June and Gene Brott, for their comments on the early drafts; Tom Frumkes, for his insights and resources; Jay and Chris, for opening my eyes to a whole new world; Jim Levine, for bringing everyone together; Tom Miller, for his deft hand and for sticking with us through the tough times; everyone in the Wiley design and production teams for making things look and sound just right; and most of all Liz, for her patience, wisdom, sense of humor, culinary skills, and just plain keeping me happy.

—Armin Brott

PART ONE

Warming and Cooling— What's Your Brain-Body Type?

Introduction

We all know what it's like to feel our very best: exhilarated, energetic, content, happy. The problem is that for most of us, moments like these are few and far between and the rest of the time we don't feel quite right.

In the past few weeks, have you:

- felt exhausted by the end of the day?
- been unable to control your food cravings?
- had a diminished sex drive?
- had periods of anxiety or anger?
- experienced feelings of helplessness or despair?
- suffered from allergies?
- had PMS or menstrual problems?
- had a tough time concentrating?
- worried that you're losing your memory?
- had trouble falling asleep or getting out of bed in the morning?
- endured chronic pain?
- struggled with addiction to cigarettes, alcohol, and/or recreational drugs?
- lost your motivation?
- just wished you felt better?

We live in the most technologically advanced society on the planet. We produce enough food to feed everyone in the world, we have access to the best medical care, and we've eradicated many of the serious illnesses that devastated previous generations. But despite all that, 20 million North Americans suffer from major depression, 70 percent have some kind of sleep difficulty, tens of millions have some form of anxiety or irritability, a huge percentage are overweight or obese, 50 million have chronic pain, and 40 million have attention deficit disorders.

Why is it that we're suffering so much?

If you have ever gone to your doctor because of any of the symptoms listed above, chances are he or she told you that you just need to relax or take a vacation or get more sleep or take some vitamins or eat better or get some exercise. You may have been told that there was nothing wrong with you at all, that your symptoms were all in your head.

Warming and Cooling

As insulting as that must have sounded, your doctor was at least partly right. Everything—from the individual cells that make up our body to the universe itself—is governed by two opposing forces: warm and cool. In the brain, those opposing forces are represented by two groups of chemicals called *neurotransmitters:* dopamine, which is warming, and serotonin, which is cooling. Together, they influence how we think and feel every second of the day and play a vital role in maintaining not only our mental but our physical well-being.

There are over a dozen different neurotransmitters running through our bodies. Each has either a warming effect (they turn something on) or a cooling one (they turn something off). Because dopamine and serotonin are the ones most representative of heating and cooling, we'll be primarily focusing on them throughout this book.

When dopamine and serotonin are properly balanced, you're healthy and you feel good inside and out. When your neurotransmitters are out of balance, you don't. And if the imbalance isn't corrected, chronic illness or disease can develop.

Your Own Natural Imbalance

We are not suggesting that neurotransmitter imbalances are the sole cause of all illness and disease. But we are saying—and we have clinical proof to back us up—that your neurotransmitters are major players in absolutely everything about you.

Each of us has his or her own ideal neurotransmitter balance. Actually, that ideal balance is a state of *imbalance,* a slight tendency toward warming or cooling. But it's precisely the right imbalance for you. It's your nature, your basic temperament, your own unique natural state of equilibrium. It's who you are when you're feeling good, when you feel most like yourself.

Your natural imbalance frames your world, determines your likes and dislikes, tolerances and abilities, and forms your personality and character. It influences every breath, every thought, every movement, and every dream. It shapes your appearance, behavior, and interests. It motivates your most important choices, including how well you get along with your friends, the job you have, your choice of marriage partner, whether or not you have children, where you live, and even the color clothes you wear.

Your natural imbalance determines your strengths and your weaknesses. If you're tilted toward warmth, you're probably alert, focused, active, energetic, attentive, engaging, confident, and fun to be with. If you're tilted toward cooling, you're probably calm, understanding, confident, capable, creative, thoughtful, unhurried, and easy to get along with.

Here's a simple test that will give you a good idea of your natural imbalance. Select the statement in each pair that comes closest to describing the way you feel.

A	B
1. I tend to be anxious rather than depressed.	I tend to be depressed more than anxious.
2. I sometimes have trouble falling or staying asleep.	I'm often tired or groggy, even after a good night's sleep.
3. I tolerate cold better than heat.	I tolerate heat better than cold.
4. I like music with a beat but sometimes I feel better after listening to some blues, soft rock, or easy listening music.	I usually listen to softer music, but sometimes I feel like hearing a rhythmic beat.
5. When I'm stressed out, I eat bread, crackers, chips, or peanuts.	When I'm stressed out, I eat chocolate, drink a Coke, or have a cup of coffee.
6. I have more trouble settling down than getting going.	I have more trouble getting going than settling down.

(continued)

7. I interrupt people and complete their sentences more than I should.	I seldom interrupt or second-guess people I'm listening to.
8. I get frustrated if things don't happen quickly enough.	I get frustrated with people or situations that cause me to rush.
9. With all that's going on, sometimes it's hard to concentrate.	Sometimes I feel like I don't have enough energy in my brain to concentrate.
10. I like to drive. Given a choice, I'll take the wheel every time.	I don't mind driving, but given a choice, I'll let someone else drive me.

If the majority of your answers were A's, you have a natural surplus of warming neurotransmitters or a cooling deficiency. If the majority of your answers were B's, you have a natural surplus of cooling neurotransmitters or a warming deficiency. We'll have a comprehensive self-evaluation quiz in chapter 2.

The problem with your natural imbalance is that it's delicate and makes you vulnerable to a constellation of symptoms and conditions. A slight cooling surplus can quickly become a warming deficiency, leaving you with a tendency toward depression, fatigue, dull thinking, memory problems, and aches and pains. And a natural warming surplus can easily turn into a cooling deficiency, leaving you anxious, restless, unable to concentrate or shut off your thoughts.

About Us

Dr. Jay Lombard is an assistant clinical professor of neurology at Cornell Medical School as well as the director of the Brain Behavior Center in Rockland County, New York, where he specializes in treating autism, ADD, ADHD, and other pediatric and adult neurobehavioral disorders. He is regarded as a leading authority on the role of supplements in psychiatric and neurological disease.

Dr. Chris Renna is the founder of LifeSpan Medicine. Having spent more than twenty years as a board-certified family practitioner, he turned his attention to the underlying causes of disease and focused his practice on preventive medicine. He returned to formal study in nutrition, metabolism, immune function, hormone regulation, mind/brain/body relationships, behavioral medicine, and the principles of DNA expression, which create either health or disease at the molecular level in response to the environment.

We met in the mid 1990s, when we were both speaking on a panel at the International Conference on Natural Therapies in Washington, D.C. Chris presented his vision of a binary brain that regulates our tendencies toward health and disease in one direction or the other. He identified the two counterbalancing systems that regulate body and mind functions: dopamine and serotonin. Chris also presented a list of physical and psychological symptoms that he attributed to imbalances of these two neurotransmitters.

Jay, a neurologist, proposed that a handful of molecules hold the key to determining the fate not only of individual cells and organs but ultimately of individuals as well. These molecules are present in every cell in our brain and body and act like reversible on-off switches that either activate or deactivate the cells. Those cells, in turn, either activate or deactivate entire organs and systems. Too many ons or too many offs could result in a system malfunction manifesting itself as a neurological or psychiatric disorder.

After listening to each other's presentations we recognized that our respective binary theories of health and disease differed only in scale. We agreed that no other factors have more influence on a person's life than his or her neurotransmitters. And we decided that if we could teach people how to understand and manage their neurotransmitters—as we'd been doing independently with our patients for years—we would be giving them a unique opportunity to change their physical, psychological, and emotional destiny. That's how this book came to be written.

How the Book Is Structured

In the first chapter we'll expand on our theory of binary—warming and cooling—systems. We'll talk about the structure of the brain and examine how each of the two hemispheres of the brain is dominated by dopamine or serotonin. You'll see how your mind and body work together. We'll talk about why so many Western physicians continue to treat the two as separate, unconnected entities. We'll also discuss some of the fascinating connections between the theories of the ancient Chinese, Greek, and Ayurvedic healers and our own high-tech understanding of neurobiology. We'll get further into the idea of balance, analyze what causes imbalance, and show how our brain is constantly trying to maintain or restore balance. We'll also talk about how the brain's attempts at rebalancing are often the opposite of what we really need.

Because every person's neurotransmitter imbalance is unique, the first step toward becoming a healthier and happier you is to take a detailed look at where you are. In chapter 2 you'll find a comprehensive test that you can take and score yourself. We've used similar tests successfully with countless patients. Once we've helped you determine your imbalance, we'll direct you to other parts of the book where we'll show you exactly how to achieve and maintain the emotional, physical, and mental balance that's perfect for you.

In chapter 3 we'll explore how warming neurotransmitters work and how imbalances influence your mind, body, and emotions and can lead to disease. In chapter 4 we'll turn the focus to cooling neurotransmitters and describe the many conditions and diseases that are caused by cooling deficiencies.

Because a large number of people have deficiencies of both warming and cooling neurotransmitters, we've included chapter 5 for a discussion of dual deficiencies.

Knowing about neurotransmitters is one thing. Putting that knowledge to use is something far more powerful and important. In chapters 6 to 8 we've created complete 28-day programs that will give you the knowledge and tools you need to naturally restore your ideal brain-body balance. Chapter 6 deals with warming deficiencies, chapter 7 with cooling, and chapter 8 with deficiencies of both. Each program includes a diet that will help you take control of your weight, vitamin and nutritional supplements to nourish your brain and body, an exercise regime to tone your body, and specific lifestyle changes that will restore your energy and help you sleep better.

Although the 28-day programs in this book will make almost everyone feel better, we recognize that a small percentage of readers won't be able to restore neurotransmitter balance by themselves. Some people are so far out of balance—often due to extreme stress or past trauma—that they can't overcome their problems on their own. For these readers and anyone else who's curious, we include suggestions for individualized hormone prescriptions and prescription medications that will go a long way toward restoring brain-body balance. We also offer background information on drugs or compounds that are effective in treating each specific imbalance.

However you do your rebalancing—whether by following the Balance Your Brain, Balance Your Life 28-day program or with the help of a trained medical professional—the benefits will be dramatic and life altering. They'll help you achieve:

- greater alertness and a more consistent energy level
- control over your weight
- freedom from food, alcohol, sugar, caffeine, or drug cravings
- a reduction of physical symptoms such as chronic pain or swelling, diminished sex drive, frequent colds or flu, migraines, PMS, or menstrual disorders
- emotional stability
- greater satisfaction and contentment with life
- decreased anger, panic, and anxiety
- improved sleep
- increased mental clarity, concentration, and decision-making ability
- a better memory
- improved mood
- elimination of depression
- improved friendships and other relationships

So read on and follow our program, and you *will* feel better in 28 days.

CHAPTER 1

The Yin and Yang of Balance, Health, and Disease

Jay had a patient, Lisa, who was a single parent trying to raise two children on her salary as a checker in a grocery store. She'd grown up in an abusive household. Just out of high school she married a policeman and moved as far away from her family as possible.

For the first few years, Lisa's marriage was good. But not long after their second son was born, her husband started coming home drunk and getting violent with her and the kids. Lisa wanted to go to counseling, but her husband refused. Instead he moved out and filed for divorce. That's when Lisa started drinking.

Her older son, who was five, developed serious emotional problems because of the divorce. And since her ex-husband refused to pay child support, Lisa and the kids were evicted from their apartment and the three of them had to move into a small studio. Lisa became horribly depressed. She stopped paying attention to her appearance, stopped exercising, put on twenty pounds, and spent most of her time drinking, watching television, and eating Pringles.

At one point, a well-meaning neighbor reported her to the Department of Social Services, who sent a caseworker to her house and threatened to place her children in foster care. Faced with the prospect of losing her children, Lisa snapped into action. On the advice of a friend she made an appointment with Jay, who determined that she had a significant cooling deficiency.

Jay prescribed Zoloft, a serotonin-increasing antidepressant, which had an immediate positive effect. But he felt that Lisa's problems would be much better dealt with in the long term by changing her lifestyle and behavior. He immediately put her on a diet like the one in the 28-day program in chapter 7, and suggested that she begin each day with some yoga or stretching, both of which increase serotonin levels. He also insisted that she get into a 12-step program, which she did.

After several months of following Jay's advice and attending regular AA meetings, Lisa had lost most of the weight she put on during her depression and had started dating. Best of all, she was feeling good enough about herself that she and Jay had begun weaning her off of the medications. Six weeks later she was completely drug-free and still feeling great.

People have been speculating for thousands of years about a connection between the mind and the body. The idea that the two are completely separate is deeply ingrained in Western culture and influences the way most contemporary physicians practice medicine and treat disease. In our system of healing, we have one group of specialists (psychologists or psychiatrists) who deal with matters of the mind, while another group (internists of all kinds) treats the body. The problem with that approach is that by treating mental and physical symptoms separately, we neglect a whole category of diseases that involve both.

There's no question that mind and body are inextricably intertwined. When our lives are in conflict or out of balance, we can literally feel it in our belly. People who are angry or depressed over a long period of time have an increased chance of suffering from heart disease. And fear can make you sweat, breathe hard, lose control of your bladder, or even die.

Most people think of "mind-body balance" as a kind of emotional-physical thing, and many of the examples we've given above—of how the body and emotions affect each other—certainly support that. But when we say mind-body balance what we really mean is *brain*-body balance, which is where the mind and the body interface. Think of it as a symphony concert. How the music sounds will depend on how well the conductor and the orchestra work together and respond to each other.

The same goes for the brain and the body. Properly balanced, they work in harmony and what happens to one has a direct impact on the other. Together, brain and body control hunger and cravings, motivate actions, temper reactions, fight infection and disease, and keep us feeling and looking our best.

What exactly are the brain and the body trying to balance? They're trying to balance two equally powerful yet opposing forces: chaos and order, excitement and inhibition, on and off, hot and cold. Some version of these two forces exists in every atom and cell in our bodies, in every muscle and nerve and organ. These forces govern our every thought and control our every action. Our lives exist in a dynamic equilibrium. Our health, our hobbies, our successes or failures in life, the relationships we have, the jobs we do, where and what we worship, and even the survival or death of single cells within our body—all depend on how well we maintain brain-body balance.

Past, Present, and Future

About 5,000 years ago the Vedic Indians were among the first to articulate the ideas that what affects the mind also affects the body and vice versa, that our emotional lives cannot be separated from our physical ones, and that health and well-being are the result of balance of mind and body. They called the two opposite forces that control us Shiva and Shakti, and they divided disease and treatment into dualities—hot and cold, strong and weak, dry and wet. Vedic physicians broke down the duality of Shiva and Shakti into three *doshas,* or life forces: Vata (air or wind), Pitta (fire or heat), and Kapha (water or liquid). Patients with too little Vata or Pitta were often described as sluggish, depressed, and having poor circulation, while patients with too much Vata or Pitta were overly ambitious, angry, and fast moving. Both sets of symptoms parallel perfectly those of dopamine deficiency or excess. Too much Kapha, on the other hand, could be responsible for a patient's apathy, lethargy, nausea, or obesity, while too little might produce chronic aches and pains, insomnia, or a constant thirst—the very complaints we'd expect to hear from patients in our offices who suffer from an excess or deficiency of serotonin.

In Chinese medicine, treatments, therapies, and methods for diagnosing illness are essentially the same today as they were 3,000 years ago. The two equal and opposite forces that are the basic principle of the universe and make up our dual nature are called yang and yin. Although the two poles are opposites, they are also mutually inseparable, each dependent on the other for growth and development. In the human mind and body, when yang and yin are not balanced, sickness occurs.

To a Chinese physician, a patient who is hot-headed, angry, flushed, an excessive risk taker, or overbearing and obnoxious would be diagnosed as having an overabundance of fire. On the other hand, a patient who was sluggish, pale, scattered, and depressed would be diagnosed as having a deficit of fire. Today, we know that both these symptoms are the result of an excess or a deficit of the warming neurotransmitters dopamine, which has a direct connection with the heart and is responsible for its rate and rhythm, and norepinephrine, which is involved in our fight-or-flight response, enabling our heart to double the volume of blood it is able to pump. During times of stress norepinephrine increases our heart rate, raises blood pressure, empties our bowels, and mobilizes stored sugar from the liver to fuel our defense, attack, or escape. If the stress goes on for too long, elevated dopamine levels can increase the risk of heart attack or stroke by making blood thicker and stickier, greatly increasing the risk of clotting in an artery.

Later the Greeks suggested that perfect mental and physical health was dependent on achieving balance among four substances called *humors,* which gave each individual his or her unique temperament, character, and strength. They called the four humors blood, phlegm, choler, and melancholy, and each matches almost perfectly with a specific neurotransmitter (NT) condition. The Greeks understood that balance would result in optimal physical and mental health. An imbalance of any one of the humors would result in disease.

Interestingly, we still use the names of all four to describe certain personality types: *sanguine* (sang is the Latin for blood) people are cheerful and have a ruddy complexion (high dopamine). Too much blood, though, and you end up manic and overaggressive. Too little and you end up apathetic and withdrawn: *phlegmatic* people are calm and unemotional (low dopamine). *Choleric* people are bad-tempered or irritable (not enough serotonin), and *melancholic* people are depressed, slow moving, and slow thinking (too much serotonin).

Western medicine has only recently been able to prove what the ancients intuited thousands of years ago. It wasn't until the 1980s that a researcher named David Felten discovered that a vast network of nerves connects the brain to blood vessels and to the major components of our immune system: bone marrow, lymph nodes, and the spleen. This discovery gave birth to a new field of medicine known as psychoneuroimmunology. The name itself reflects the connection between the psychological, neurological, and immune systems.

The similarities between ancient healing systems and our own knowledge of NTs go far beyond the metaphorical. Dopamine really *is* about heat. It acts directly on the *hypothalamus,* the body's thermostat located in the brain, and helps us maintain our body temperature. Dopamine also regulates heat indirectly, stimulating our metabolism at a hormonal and cellular level. It turns on our immune system and regulates our sexual inclinations, firing up our passions. It activates receptors in the heart that elevate blood pressure and make it beat faster. Without dopamine, our heart cells wouldn't contract, our muscles wouldn't move, and our immune cells would refuse to battle invaders.

Conversely, serotonin really *is* about cooling and slowing things down. In Chinese medicine, water counterbalances the force of fire. That's exactly what serotonin does, keeping the dopamine-fired immune system from overheating and attacking itself. It also slows the release of adrenalin, which moderates the amount of blood that flows to the heart during the fight-or-flight response. Like water, serotonin is necessary for survival, and like water, it flows through us, nurturing and cooling the brain and body. It regulates our moods and emotions, heightens our senses, and helps us adapt to new surroundings and experiences. Serotonin's influence goes far beyond the psychological. It influences brain growth and development, cardiovascular and reproductive function, sleep, dietary choices, body temperature, and the perception of pain.

Every branch of modern Western medicine is designed around the twin concepts of equal and opposite forces and of imbalance being the cause of disease and illness. In this book we'll be referring to these two forces as *warming* and *cooling* or *hot* and *cold.*

Cardiologists, for example, treat abnormalities of the heart. The heart that beats too fast (too hot) is slowed with medication. The heart that beats too slowly (too cold) is sped up with a different medication. Blood pressure that's too high must be lowered and pressure that's too low must be raised. Oncologists treat cancer, which is the result of cells that grow too fast (heat), and at the same time try to stimulate an immune system that isn't working fast enough (cool). An endocrinologist might treat diabetes caused by too little insulin (too cold) or metabolic syndrome caused by too much insulin (too hot). And the emergency room physician lowers the body temperature of a feverish patient (one whose temperature is too high) and warms the hypothermic patient (one whose temperature is too low). Each of these medical specialists dedicates himself or herself to recognizing the symptoms of imbalance based on the organizing principle of dual recip-rocal forces.

Not all imbalances are severe enough to be life-threatening or even to be called a disease. Minor imbalances are responsible for most of the conditions that affect us every day—the aches and pains, headaches, back and neck stiffness, infections, rashes, fatigue, excessive weight gain or loss, insomnia, hormonal imbalances, and mood problems such as irritability, anxiety, depression, hostility, and aggression.

Unfortunately, there is a disconnect in the Western medical com-munity between doctors who take care of minds and those who take care of bodies. A psychiatrist who prescribes a serotonin-enhancing drug for a patient's depression and underlying feelings of hostility and anger and the cardiologist who treats the same patient's angina may never speak to each other—even though both symptoms are undoubt-edly related to the same NT imbalance and should be treated together. A recent study, for example, showed that heart patients who were treated with serotonin-enhancing drugs were 40 percent less likely to die of heart-related illness than those who weren't.

If the patient were seeing a Chinese or Ayurvedic medical practi-tioner, he or she would probably make the connection between all the symptoms. But we in the West need to learn about these connections and incorporate the knowledge into our medical treatments and daily lives.

What Is Balance?

Let's take a minute to consider what balance actually is. Until now we've talked about balance as if our objective is a perfect, exactly equal, fifty-fifty blend. As wonderful as that idea sounds, true balance is far more subtle than that.

Each of us has a unique ideal balance. What it takes to make you feel and look your best may have little in common with what it takes to get the same results for someone else. The balance that's right for you depends on your individual genes, your body chemistry, what your mother was eating when she was pregnant with you, your personality, temperament, lifestyle, living situation, and so on. It also depends on your own personal definition of feeling your best.

There's really no such thing as perfect balance. The two forces of warm and cool are constantly evolving. Neither can exist without the other. They work together, influencing and being influenced by each other, creating and being created by each other. It's a never-ending flow. Wherever you find one, you'll find the other as well.

The bottom line is that the struggle to get *close* to a state of balance that is perfect and unique for each one of us is what keeps us alive and well. The closer we get, the better we feel, which is why we keep chasing after it. But we're not always perfect in our attempts. If we overshoot in one direction or don't respond to something in the other, the balance shifts and we feel sick or we develop symptoms of disease.

Our brain tries to maintain balance between the two, sometimes unpredictable, forces of warming and cooling by meeting every force with an equal and opposite one. It's a tough job, aggravated by our poor eating habits, stress, lack of physical activity, pollution, social isolation, substance abuse, the temperature outside, the bad or good news we just heard, even the length of time since our last meal. The constant flow of internal and external stimuli makes it difficult for us to remain level.

Although most of us are out of balance most of the time, we're not *so* far out that our brain, which contains our own internal righting mechanism, can't catch us and straighten us out, restoring us to our natural disposition. If the righting mechanism works, we have a smooth flight and we don't even notice the tiny corrections that are happening every second. If it doesn't work, our levels of warming and cooling get so far out of alignment that we experience turbulence.

The Two Hemispheres of the Brain

The human brain is uniquely organized into two hemispheres. The left is rational and objective and is dominated by dopamine. It thrives and feels at home in a world that is ordered, predictable, and secure. It's assertive, activity oriented, and verbally expressive. Had the Chinese thought in terms of left and right brain, they would have called the left side yang, the fire side, the side that governs warmth, brightness, expansiveness, movement, and agitation. The left brain is responsible for coherent thought. It is reality, wakefulness, concrete science, and Western rationalism.

Primarily governed by serotonin, the right hemisphere's personality is the exact opposite—emotional, feeling, and subjective. The Chinese would have called it yin, because it is dark, receding, contracting, and cool. The right brain deals with the amorphous. It houses our fantasies and dreams and the vestiges of our primitive unconscious. The right brain deals with the aspects of our lives and environment that are mysterious, unknown, and chaotic. And since all of these are potential threats, the right brain exerts an inhibitory influence on our behavior and our thoughts.

Neurotransmitters and Mind and Body

The communication between the brain's left and right hemispheres and between them and every other cell in your body takes place over a network of billions of miles of interconnected nerves. The messengers that make all this communication possible are our neurotransmitters. They are the language that forms the infinite number of communication feedback loops that link our brain, body, organs, systems, and cells. Working together with the immune and endocrine (hormone) systems, our neurotransmitters sense and perceive everything we are and everything we know. They instantly convey information from every part of the brain to every other part, and from the brain throughout the rest of the body. They enable us to live and interact in our world, to think, feel, see, hear, form memories, show emotion, love, and breathe. In a sense, our neurotransmitters are us.

For the most part in this book we'll be dealing with correcting deficiencies—it's generally easier to give you something you don't have rather than take away something you have too much of. Every once in a while, though, a condition is actually caused by an excess of one particular neurotransmitter as opposed to a deficit of the corresponding one. In those cases, the cure usually requires reducing the excess rather than boosting the deficit. We'll talk about those situations when we get to them.

There's no question that on the most fundamental level, we are the bodily manifestations of our NTs. Imagine that you're walking down the street when you hear a tremendous crash. Your brain instantly releases a tiny bit of dopamine, which speeds up your pulse, dilates your pupils, tenses your muscles, and gets you ready to handle what might be a dangerous situation. Your neurotransmitter balance has just tilted toward dopamine. After you survey the situation and come to the conclusion that the noise wasn't anything to be afraid of, your brain releases some serotonin to calm you back down. Now your balance is tilted toward serotonin.

The same kind of thing is happening inside us millions of times a second. Every breath we take, sight we see, thought we have, step we take, bite we chew, conversation we have, place we go, book we read stimulates the release of certain NTs. The result is a never-ending process of oscillation between dopamine and serotonin.

If it weren't for the brain's remarkable ability to instantly adapt to its ever-changing environment by making tiny corrections, we couldn't make it through a day alive. Most of the time the brain's response to NT imbalance has the desired effect. But when the imbalance becomes too severe, or something interferes with the brain's ability to regulate NT production and release, we end up with disease or illness.

In the next chapter you'll take a quiz that will educate you about your own natural balances and imbalances. Later you'll learn what to do about them.

CHAPTER 2

Your Personal Brain-Body Type Assessment

The first step is to pay attention to how you're feeling. You probably aren't very aware of your body most of the time—unless you're not feeling as well as you'd like or you're unable to do what you want. It's precisely that sort of dissatisfaction or discomfort that will give you the incentive you need to make the changes that will get you feeling your best. To start the process, we'd like you to take the test that begins on the next page.

In the test that follows, read each statement and score it as follows:

- 0 points if the statement is not true at all or doesn't apply to you
- 1 point if the statement is true some of the time
- 2 points if the statement is true most or all of the time

Once you've analyzed your results, we'll refer you to either the warming or cooling sections of this book, depending on your particular results. There you'll find a thorough description of how that neurotransmitter works and symptoms related to imbalance.

THE BALANCE YOUR BRAIN, BALANCE YOUR LIFE TEST

1. I've had a lot of intimate relationships, but they never seem to last.
2. I have a tough time getting used to new routines.
3. It takes me a long time to get sexually aroused.
4. When I finally make a decision, I spend a lot of time second-guessing and wondering whether I did the right thing.
5. I love going to new places and adapt right away.
6. I frequently lack self-confidence and doubt my abilities.
7. I'm just not motivated to exercise. I want to, but I just can't seem to make myself do it.
8. I have excessive fears or worries, persistent phobias, or nervousness.
9. I have a tough time getting organized and completing tasks.
10. My desktop is so neat that my coworkers sometimes joke that my office looks unoccupied.
11. I have trouble getting up in the morning.
12. I've been diagnosed with an autoimmune disorder.
13. Once I make a decision, I'm on to other things.
14. I'm very concerned about my appearance and worry a lot about my many physical flaws.
15. I watch more than three hours of television every day.
16. The thought of having something old or moldy in my fridge really bothers me.
17. My mental reaction time is slow.
18. I carry most of my weight around my middle.
19. I absolutely can't stand it when things don't go my way.
20. I prefer quiet places without lots of bright lights.
21. I have been careless on more than one occasion about the person I have sex with.
22. Songs and jingles often get stuck in my head.
23. I have no idea why people make such a big deal out of messy desks. I know I have a lot of piles, but I know exactly where everything is.

24. When I go to a party I don't socialize much. I tend to sit by myself or stay close to people I know.

25. If someone cuts me off in traffic, I'll pull ahead and cut them off.

26. I have more trouble relaxing than getting going.

27. I have low blood pressure.

28. I'm extremely cautious and don't like to take risks.

29. I smoke cigarettes.

30. I'd rather stay home than go out.

31. I get angry easily but I calm down quickly.

32. I fidget a lot.

33. I have a slow physical reaction time and I feel clumsy a lot of the time.

34. I have problems falling and staying asleep.

35. I tend to be sad or depressed a lot of the time.

36. People tell me I'm thin but I never believe them.

37. If I'm assembling something, I don't pay much attention to the directions and I sometimes end up with extra pieces.

38. I prefer mild foods or no seasonings at all.

39. I'm frequently constipated.

40. I'm shy and sometimes withdrawn.

41. I frequently feel cold when everyone around me is warm.

42. I spend a long time considering all the options before making a decision.

43. I have a learning disability now or had one when I was a child.

44. I like the bedroom cool and sometimes throw the covers off.

45. I think or know that I have ADD.

46. I've been told I have hyperthyroidism.

47. I can sleep through anything.

48. My weight fluctuates dramatically.

49. I have a family history of problems with blood sugar regulation, hypoglycemia, or diabetes.

50. When it comes to the weekend, I like to have everything planned out in advance.

51. I drink more than three cups of coffee a day.

52. Everything is organized in my closet. All the pants are together, all the shirts are together, and the hangers face the same way.

53. I have difficulties absorbing new information.

54. I don't have as much appetite as other people.

55. I'm not as interested in sex as I used to be.

56. I get more angry at myself than at others.

57. I frequently feel lethargic, tired, or bored.

58. I have very dry skin.

59. No matter how hard I try, I always seem to get to places late.

60. I get anxious, hostile, or angry right before my period.

61. I'm frequently congested or have lots of allergies.

62. I'm sometimes tired and restless at the same time.

63. If I get really angry, I might get into a physical fight.

64. Once I get a thought in my head, I think about it over and over and over.

65. I carry my weight evenly, even on my limbs and torso.

66. I'm worried about my health and make a lot of medical appointments.

67. I've changed jobs more than five times in the last three years.

68. My total cholesterol is below 150.

69. I suffer from recurrent infections.

70. I sometimes feel dizzy.

71. I have had dreams of falling.

72. I crave carbohydrates and sweets.

73. It takes a lot to bring me to tears.

74. I have incredibly vivid dreams, sometimes nightmares.

75. I have a family history of cancer.

76. My moods change constantly and unexpectedly.

77. I have more trouble getting going than relaxing.

78. My mind races when trying to fall asleep.

79. I have high cholesterol.

80. If someone cuts me off in traffic, I won't do anything, but I'll be angry about it for hours afterward.

81. I perspire excessively.

82. I need the security of a long-term relationship and often stay even if I'm not happy.

83. I get excited easily and I find myself taking unnecessary risks.

84. I suffer from premature ejaculation.

85. I have osteoarthritis.

86. I frequently worry that I've done something wrong even when I know I haven't.

87. I sometimes feel confused or as if my brain is in a fog.

88. Before the stock market crash I had most of my investments in bonds or very conservative funds.

89. I don't really care what anyone thinks about how I look.

90. I have a family history of heart disease.

91. I have things in my refrigerator that are past their expiration date or moldy.

92. When I'm most depressed, I sometimes think about suicide.

93. I have a family history of drug addiction.

94. I'm a neat freak and can't stand messiness or disorder.

95. I often make off-the-cuff decisions and don't really consider the consequences.

96. I have a ruddy (flushed-looking) complexion, blush easily, and/or get skin rashes.

97. My memory's not what it used to be. I sometimes find things I've misplaced in very strange places.

98. I like painkillers or tranquilizers such as Valium, Xanax, and Ativan.

99. I never feel rested no matter how much sleep I get.

100. I can work out for an hour but I never seem to perspire.

101. I'm extremely confident—sometimes so much that I overestimate my abilities.

102. I suffer from high blood pressure, hypertension, palpitations, angina, or cardiac rhythm problems.

103. I'm the life of the party.

104. I feel a lot better about sex after a couple of drinks.

105. I rarely remember my dreams.

106. I'm hypersensitive to smell; perfumes and strong odors really bother me.

107. I crave fried foods, meats, or salty foods.

108. When I don't get what I want, I almost never complain.

109. I often have trouble finding the right words when speaking.

110. I have chronic pain, fibromyalgia, or sciatica.

111. I can eat any kind of food in any combination and I never feel bad.

112. I often need a good stiff drink to help me settle down.

113. I don't worry about my health at all—what will be will be. I haven't been to see a doctor in years.

114. I'm slow to anger, but it takes me a long time to settle back down.

115. I have chronic fatigue syndrome or think I do.

116. I frequently feel warm when everyone around me is cold.

117. I'm easily distracted and sometimes have a hard time paying attention or concentrating.

118. I get frequent diarrhea.

119. I get depressed and puffy and have tender breasts right before my period.

120. If I'm assembling something, I read the directions very carefully and double-check each step.

121. The clothes in my closet are all mixed up, hanging in random order.

122. I tend to be anxious or nervous.

123. I love bright, loud places.

124. Once I've learned something, it's hard for me to change the way I do things.

125. I get more angry at others than at myself.

126. I think or know that I have obsessive-compulsive disorder (OCD).

127. I crave chocolate.

128. I grind my teeth or have Temporomandibular Disorder (TMD).

129. When it comes to the weekend, I prefer to do things spontaneously and not make plans.

130. I have more than three alcoholic drinks a day.

131. I tend to be on the heavy side and have trouble losing weight.

132. If something bad happens to me, I can't seem to get it out of my head.

133. I've been told I have hypothyroidism.

134. I'm never late and I get very annoyed if anyone else is.

135. I like to sleep with lots of covers.

136. I've had seizures or been diagnosed with epilepsy.

137. I sometimes have a swollen face or ankles.

138. I cry easily.

139. I like my foods hot and spicy.

140. I sometimes get migraines or experience regular tension headaches.

141. I find it difficult to think abstractly and had trouble with things like geometry in school.

142. I have had dreams of floods or drowning.

143. I've had hives, cystic acne, or frequent fever blisters or cold sores.

144. I've had the same job for twenty years. I don't really like it, but I don't want to make waves.

145. I'm a little overweight but I don't really care.

146. I tend to hold a grudge for a long time.

147. I'd rather go out than stay home.

148. I almost never get sick.

149. I'm sometimes absent-minded or forgetful and have trouble remembering appointments and names.

150. I suffer from asthma.

Calculating Your Score

1. Add up the total number of points you scored on the odd-numbered questions only.
    a. If you scored 40 or more, you have a definite warming neurotransmitter deficiency. After you've carefully read chapter 3, implement the 28-day plan in chapter 6.
    b. If you scored 25–40, you have a minor warming deficiency. In order to keep yourself from slipping into a more severe deficiency, we suggest that you read chapter 3 carefully and then implement the 28-day plan in chapter 6.

2. Add up the total amount of points you scored on the even-numbered questions only.
    a. If you scored 40 or more, you have a definite cooling neurotransmitter deficiency. After you've carefully read chapter 4, implement the 28-day plan in chapter 7.
    b. If you scored 25–40 points, you have a minor cooling deficiency. In order to keep yourself from slipping into a more severe deficiency, we suggest that you read chapter 4 carefully, and implement the 28-day plan in chapter 7.

3. If you scored fewer than 25 points on the even-numbered questions *and* fewer than 25 points on the odd-numbered questions, congratulations! You're doing fine. But keep in mind that neurotransmitter levels change every day in response to everything that goes on within and around you. If you stop feeling as good as you want to, take the test again. And read the rest of this book so you can understand the mind-body connection better.

4. If you scored more than 40 points on the even-numbered questions *and* more than 40 points on the odd-numbered questions, you have a deficiency of both warming and cooling neurotransmitters. You need to read all of the following chapters and implement our action steps.

The overwhelming majority of people will respond extremely well to the appropriate 28-day plan. But occasionally we need to explore more advanced methods of diagnosing and rebalancing. We'll discuss a number of approaches you can follow under your doctor's supervision, such as prescription medications and hormones, as well as others he or she may not be aware of.

But one thing is certain: No matter how far out of balance you are, you *will* be able to make the changes you need. The results will amaze you. You'll be happier and more alert, sleep better, have more energy and a better memory, take control of your weight, and feel more satisfied with life.

CHAPTER 3

Are You Too Cool?

How Warming Deficiencies Affect Your Mind and Body

Carol was a star athlete in high school and attended a well-known university on a four-year golf scholarship. At twenty-six, she was one of the youngest players in the LPGA competing for hundreds of thousands of dollars in prize money and lucrative product endorsement contracts. Although she had an athlete's body, muscular and fit, she looked tired and worn down when she first arrived in Chris's office.

Carol suspected that she had chronic fatigue and/or fibromyalgia, but when she shared her suspicions with her doctors they scoffed. She read a number of books that offered quick cures, but nothing worked.

Carol also complained that she was having problems concentrating. While taking Chris through her medical history, she had trouble remembering basic details about her illness. At one point she couldn't remember the name of the doctor who had treated her for months—even though she had seen him two weeks before consulting Chris.

Carol was bright, mature, and determined. Still, she was anxious and worried that her illness would ruin everything she'd worked for. Her diet was fairly healthy, but because of her tiredness, she'd started consuming caffeinated drinks and high-sugar foods in an attempt to boost her energy levels. She used to exercise regularly but had given it up because every time she worked out she felt sick and achy. Carol slept eight or nine hours a night but always woke up feeling that she needed another hour or two in bed.

When she first got sick, Carol started taking a multivitamin plus some additional vitamin B for energy. Every time she heard or read about a supplement or vitamin or mineral or herb compound that promised to restore energy, she added it to her regimen. By the time she met with Chris she was taking over ninety pills every day!

Her history was a classic warming deficiency, and lab tests revealed low levels of antioxidants and low levels of three hormones—testosterone, thyroid, and human growth hormone. This last one was especially surprising, given her age and exceptional physical abilities.

The first thing Chris did was take Carol off all the pills. After three days of cold turkey, she said she felt a little less pain but even more tired than before. Chris then started Carol on a 28-day program similar to the one explained in chapter 6: a medium-to-high-protein diet to provide the amino acids and vitamins she needed to increase her dopamine levels, low-intensity exercise—just enough to produce a sweat, no more—every day for two weeks, and restricted her sleep to a maximum of eight hours per day with no naps. More protein, more intense exercise, and more stimulating herbs and supplements might have helped Carol's energy levels, but they also might have triggered an immune system response that would have increased her pain. She needed to be patient.

Within a month, Carol had shown great improvement. She was up to three to four pain-free workouts a week. With every day, Carol gradually began to feel more like her old self. After three months she no longer needed to take hormones or restrict her workouts or sleep habits. Within six months she was off prescription drugs and was able to return to the LPGA tour. Today she's playing better than ever and believes that following the program enabled her to avoid a career-ending problem.

You remember what it feels like to be at the top of your game, don't you? Your thoughts come quickly and clearly, you're energetic, upbeat, assertive, and decisive; you feel healthy and fit and attractive. What you're experiencing when you feel this way is the focus, concentration, and exhilaration that comes when you've got high, balanced levels of warming and cooling neurotransmitters in your brain. Unfortunately, those wonderful feelings don't usually last nearly as long as you'd like them to. The rest of the time—which is a lot of the time—your levels of dopamine and other warming neurotransmitters are low and life isn't nearly as pleasant. You may:

- be depressed . . . or manic or anxious
- feel lethargic and apathetic . . . or severely angry and unable to handle frustration
- have no sense of adventure . . . or be prone to taking excessive risks
- have little or no sex drive . . . or be obsessed with sex
- be unable to concentrate . . . or have memory problems
- suffer from high cholesterol, carbohydrate and fat cravings, hay fever, muscle weakness, fatigue, drug addiction or alcoholism, low or high blood pressure, ADD, and even cancer

Although some of these symptoms may sound contradictory, they're all governed by four warming neurotransmitters that work together closely: dopamine, norepinephrine, glutamate, and acetylcholine. However, their origins, distribution networks, effects, and the symptoms they produce, can be subtly, or not so subtly, different. For the remainder of this chapter, we'll refer to the four of them together as *warming neurotransmitters* or *warming NTs* except when we need to discuss a specific one separately.

Our warming neurotransmitters play a role in nearly every aspect of our lives. They move us to act, keep life from being physically painful, and reward us for taking chances. When inaction, pain, and indecisiveness make life intolerable, these warming NTs make it better. Together, they control our:

- emotions and mood
- behavior
- desires (including our sexual desires, ambitions, and even choice of foods and clothing)
- critical brain functions, including memory
- voluntary and involuntary movement
- ability to enjoy life

Your mind knows intuitively when something is out of balance, and it often directs your body to do exactly what needs to be done to correct the problem and restore your natural disposition. Reaching for that cup of coffee when you're feeling drowsy first thing in the morning (or afternoon), sitting down to a high-protein bacon-and-eggs breakfast or ordering a cheeseburger for lunch, and pulling the covers over your head last thing at night are all instinctive ways you stimulate your warming neurotransmitters. The same goes for that light stretching you do to work the morning stiffness out of your muscles. But not all imbalances are as easily self-diagnosed (and self-treated), and sometimes the things we do to try to rebalance ourselves are precisely the wrong things to do. Reaching for a third cup of coffee in the morning, for example, might seem like a good idea, even to our unconscious. The brain might think, Hey, it worked before. . . . But you can only go to the caffeine well so often before it runs dry. Caffeine releases a chemical inside our cells that increases energy just as the warming NTs do. The difference is that when the chemical is stimulated by warming neurotransmitters, it gets replenished. But caffeine depletes it. Caffeine also exhausts the levels of micronutrients needed by the brain, which results in the classic caffeine tremor.

If the mind and body are two halves of the same whole, neurotransmitters are the glue that keeps the pieces together. Using sophisticated scientific methods, we now know exactly how most NTs function. Let's take a look at where our warming NTs come from and some of the ways they work—independently and together—to affect our minds, emotions, bodies, and behavior.

Dopamine and Norepinephrine

Dopamine is produced from the amino acid tyrosine in the *substantia nigra,* an area of the brain that controls the body's movements and expresses the mind's moods through action. The substantia nigra is located at the center of the brain and acts as a command post from which dopamine sends messages to receptors located throughout the brain.

As it wends its way through the brain, dopamine breaks down into a number of other chemical compounds, the most important of which is norepinephrine, the primary neurotransmitter involved in wakefulness and alertness. At first glance, norepinephrine seems nearly the same as dopamine. Chemically, they are extremely close. The enzyme *dopamine hydroxylase* (DBH) converts dopamine into norepinephrine in one step. But norepinephrine is more stimulatory; it drives the brain and helps dopamine deliver its signals hard and fast. It keeps us alert and oriented, makes us get up and go, lets us multitask and moves us toward accomplishment and order. Norepinephrine, the first by-product of dopamine, is the warming chemical that keeps us going. It's all logic and business and action.

Dopamine, on the other hand, is fun. It fills us with desire, gives us a sense of optimism and possibility, motivates us to take the kind of risks we need to keep life interesting, urges us to try new and enjoyable things, and gives us our appetite. It helps us manage our emotions as well as integrate feelings and movement, which means our bodies can have a physical reaction to emotion: we jump when we're happy, freeze when we're frightened, run when we're threatened. Most importantly, though, dopamine is the source of the highest pleasures the brain can perceive, and it gives us a reward every time we do something it thinks is right. But, as with everything, moderation is the key. The pursuit of dopamine-created feelings of pleasure is often the force behind addictive behavior. We'll talk more about that a little later in this chapter.

Dopamine is responsible for what's called the *affective component* of your memory—the part that makes you believe an event is worthwhile enough to reserve a sufficient amount of space in the part of the brain where memories are stored. Just think about your most vivid memories: the first time you had sex or what you were doing when you heard that JFK was shot or hijacked planes were flown into the World Trade Center. A deficit of dopamine in the *prefrontal cortex* of the brain can have the same effects on memory as an injury to that same area of the brain.

Disruptions to dopamine production in the *limbic system* (which helps control our movement and mood) can have a number of possible physical and psychological ramifications, including major depressive disorder, attention deficit disorder (ADD), attention deficit hyperactivity disorder (ADHD), and anxiety. Our limbic system is linked with our endocrine system, which controls hormone production and influences the growth and production of cells and neurons.

Norepinephrine is responsible for conscious registration of external stimuli. In a number of studies, animals with a malfunctioning norepinephrine system have less efficient mechanisms for learning, so they're more easily distracted and hardly interested in anything new or unusual. Norepinephrine stimulates the brain's wakefulness center, which is why high levels are associated with anxiety and arousal and low levels with dullness and lack of energy and motivation.

Brandon's Story:
Warming Deficiency and Libido

A forty-three-year-old male nurse, Brandon had been battling depression for most of his adult life. He'd taken most of the serotonin-enhancing antidepressants and had success each time, pulling him out of the dark hole he felt he was in and making life more enjoyable. The problem was that each of those drugs produced at least one sexual problem, including loss of libido, difficulty achieving or maintaining an erection, or ejaculatory failure. So Brandon took himself off the drugs and slipped back into his pit.

As in many cases like this, Brandon wasn't the only one affected by his depression-or-sex dilemma. His wife found it hard to deal with either the depressed but sexually active Brandon, or the not depressed but uninterested-in-sex Brandon, and the marriage was in trouble.

Brandon was initially reluctant to add another prescription medication while on SSRIs, so Jay prescribed ginseng. It increases warming neurotransmitters and nitric oxide production— the same thing that Viagra does. After a few days on the SSRI/ginseng combination, Brandon noticed that his erections were much firmer. But his libido was still very low. After some encouragement from his wife and Jay, Brandon reluctantly agreed to take Wellbutrin, a dopamine-enhancing drug. Last time Jay saw Brandon and his wife, they were arm in arm and appeared to be doing well.

Acetylcholine

Acetylcholine has been around longer than people have, and there's evidence that it is a major player in the evolution of life as we know it. Acetylcholine is involved in the function, structure, division, protection, and cell membrane development of a variety of life forms. Scientists have detected acetylcholine in worms, bacteria, yeast, algae, and even some plants. The acetylcholine system is also intimately involved in attention, cognitive performance, and glucose utilization in the brain, and it enhances the release of a number of other neurotransmitters, including dopamine, norepinephrine, and glutamate.

Acetylcholine is a by-product of *choline,* an essential nutrient involved in neuromuscular activity. It's also the predominant brain chemical of the mind, acting as a kind of cognitive fertilizer, keeping brain cells from dying prematurely and literally providing us with food for thought. It allows us to digest, absorb, process, assimilate, and remember new information. Experiments have shown that low-choline diets reduce cognitive ability and motor function. Properly balanced, acetylcholine enables us to learn, improves our memory, and makes us smarter. Without it our minds are dull. We can't concentrate or organize our thoughts, no new memories can be formed, and old ones disappear—symptoms typically associated with Alzheimer's disease and other forms of dementia.

Acetylcholine is the primary warming neurotransmitter in the brain, and it plays a critical role in memory and learning. Drugs that block acetylcholine in the brain result in impaired attention, amnesia, and memory problems. New experiences and sensory inputs stimulate one particular set of acetylcholine receptors. That in turn increases the products of *brain-derived neurotrophic factor* (BDNF), which fertilizes brain cells, protecting them, preventing premature death, and helping the brain repair itself. This actually causes physical changes in the brain that make further learning possible. There's evidence that Alzheimer's and Parkinson's diseases are both related to a lack of BDNF.

Acetylcholine breaks down memories into tiny pieces and stores them in the neurons of the brain, sort of like how your computer divides your data and stores it all over your hard drive. When you're learning something or acquiring a new memory, your acetylcholine levels increase. But a deficiency of acetylcholine means that the tiny fragments of memory can't reconnect with one another. Memories are lost or at least unretrievable.

A deficit of acetylcholine is often associated with the following symptoms:

* problems finding the right word
* difficulty absorbing new information/loss of short-term memory
* difficulty focusing
* difficulty thinking abstractly
* indecision
* forgetfulness
* problems with geographical orientation

- trouble recalling dreams
- learning disability
- Alzheimer's disease

Increasing the amount of acetylcholine in the brain improves the ability to focus, pay attention, and create memories—especially emotional memories. Many drugs used to treat ADD work by stimulating dopamine release, which in turn triggers acetylcholine release, resulting in increased attention span. Some researchers believe that stimulating this same mechanism is responsible for many of the focus- and memory-related improvements seen in Alzheimer's patients who are treated with acetylcholine-enhancing drugs.

Glutamate

Glutamate is a product of *glutamic acid.* Technically, it's an amino acid, but it acts like a neurotransmitter. Glutamate comes in two basic flavors: the kind in your body and the kind in your brain. On an average day, you probably consume 10 to 20 grams of glutamate, and your body produces about 50 grams more. Your body stores a lot of that extra glutamate and uses it to regulate your metabolism—you've probably got about four pounds of it stored in your kidneys, liver, and muscles.

Glutamate is one of the primary warming neurotransmitters in your brain. It's found in every cell in our brain and is critical to all of our mental, sensory, motor, and emotional functions. It moves nutrients from where they are to where they're needed and strengthens connections between brain cells. It quickly and efficiently transmits messages throughout the brain by flooding it with the materials it needs to organize new thoughts, store them, and recall them on demand. It's critical to our ability to perceive pain. Glutamate in the brain is a good thing. The only problem is that too much of it can overstimulate cells, resulting in conditions such as stroke, epilepsy, bipolar disease, dementia, chronic pain, migraines, and ALS, more often called Lou Gehrig's disease.

Glutamate facilitates the communication of all information between neurons, which means it's involved in every step—encoding, storing, and retrieving memories. When glutamate receptors are stimulated, they release calcium into the surrounding brain cells. This releases a pro-inflammatory fatty acid called *arachidonic acid,* as well as a number of specialized proteins that excite individual cells and make them receptive to incoming information. If an experience is worth remembering or is repeated often enough, glutamate literally reshapes your brain, creating new synaptic pathways that enable you to recall the event.

Warming Deficiencies and Your Mind and Body

Your medical history is the most important diagnostic tool you and your practitioner have. And in general, your symptoms provide the most important part of that history. This section is devoted to a discussion of how a warming neurotransmitter deficiency may affect your mind, body, and behavior. But before we start, please remember these three things:

1. Unless you're a hypochondriac or very imbalanced, you're not going to have all of the symptoms described here.
2. Not all warming deficiencies are the same. Yours may be affecting your mood, while someone else's may be affecting memory, and yet another person's may be causing Parkinson's disease.
3. Your mind and your body are connected to and influenced by each other. All the subsystems of your mind and body are interconnected as well, each reflecting and affecting the others, each like a hologram, identical to but smaller than the larger system. The struggle for balance that's taking place in your brain is also playing out in your emotions, your hormones, your intellect, and everywhere else. The symptoms of that imbalance may simply be more obvious in certain areas than in others.

Warming neurotransmitters play a variety of roles in your ability to focus, pay attention, learn, and create memories, and in your brain's overall ability to function. Symptoms of warming deficits include:

- inattentiveness and problems concentrating
- scattered or foggy thinking, spaciness, or forgetfulness
- an absence of dreams or dreams of falling
- reduced speed of information processing and capacity for abstract thinking
- difficulty acquiring and retaining new information
- impaired attention span and ability to focus

Depression and Warming Deficiency

Depression is a very common condition that can be caused by a deficiency of either warming or cooling neurotransmitters—and in some cases by a deficiency of both. Both types of depression feature feelings of emptiness, guilt, and worthlessness. But there are some significant differences.

Cooling-deficiency depression is marked by anxieties, insomnia, decreased appetite, and panic attacks. We discuss this type of depression in chapter 4. That means that you, like many of the warming-deficient patients who come into our office, will have some or all of the following core symptoms:

- low energy, fatigue, and/or lack of motivation
- looking dull and bored
- excessive need for sleep
- no sense of adventure or pain
- being quiet and unengaging
- being extremely introverted and withdrawn
- a decline in, or absence of, nurturing behavior
- feelings of apathy
- loss of libido
- inability to take pleasure in life
- postpartum blues or depression

The common denominator uniting these symptoms—and the most common complaint among people with a warming deficiency—is fatigue. Fatigue is the biological condition that results from an insufficient supply of energy or energy-producing ability. That, of course, has a major influence on our overall sense of well-being. Disturbances in well-being, however minor, are reflected in our thoughts, emotions, appearance, and motivations or choices. Well-being comes about from the interaction of the warming neurotransmitters and their ability to counterbalance the effects of the cooling NTs. The cascade of warming activity produced by the interactions of dopamine, norepinephrine, acetylcholine, and glutamate is the source of "feeling good." When warming NTs are out of balance and deficient—whether it's because of genetic tendencies, stress, environmental factors, viruses, bacteria, parasites, or simply aging—we feel tired and depressed or, at the very least, not as well as we'd like to.

Richard's Story:
Warming Deficiency and Depression

Richard, fifty-nine, was a partner in a major law firm. He was well respected and did quite well financially. But despite his successes, Richard had battled depression on and off for most of his life. On his first visit with Jay, Richard described himself as feeling "weighed down" by life and as being in a "cold, damp pit." He was excessively tired and needed 10 to 11 hours of sleep a night but never felt rested. He was overweight, bored with his marriage, apathetic, and unmotivated, and couldn't take pleasure in anything. At work, he often felt "frozen" and had a terrible time making decisions.

Over the years, Richard's psychiatrist had prescribed a variety of different antidepressants, but because they were boosting his cooling neurotransmitters, they just made him even sleepier.

Jay started Richard on the 28-day program described in chapter 7, which he augmented with the dopamine-enhancing drug Wellbutrin. Within the first week Richard reported significant improvements in daily energy and his quality of sleep. By the end of the 28 days he had lost 12 pounds, complained less of being frozen and weighed down, and generally felt like a new man. His energy and confidence were restored, and he once again felt as if his life was in balance.

ADD/ADHD and Warming Deficiency

Tom came to see Jay at the urging of his parents. At age twenty, he seemed to be floundering. He was still living at home, wasn't working, and had no direction in his life. Tom and his parents fought a lot, usually about his chain smoking, the endless hours he spent in front of the television, or his refusal to help out around the house in any way. He'd recently lost his driver's license because of a DUI. In his first meeting with Jay, Tom complained of being constantly bored, not having any motivation, and being too easily distracted.

As a child, Tom was speech and reading delayed. He was forgetful and disorganized, and his homework—on the rare occasions when he turned it in—was barely legible. He always seemed to be in trouble and was even suspended several times. He struggled just as much in high school and dropped out at the beginning of his senior year.

His parents helped him get a job, but he lost it after a few weeks. Other jobs followed, but they never seemed to last more than a month. Tom was often late, didn't complete his work, and argued with his boss and coworkers.

An EEG showed significant slowing in Tom's frontal lobes—the kind of activity typically seen in children and adults with ADD and/or ADHD. Other tests determined that Tom's symptoms were being caused by deficiencies in both dopamine and acetylcholine.

Jay started Tom on a program to modify his diet, but Tom could never seem to follow the directions and stay on the plan. With help from his parents, however, Tom was able to take a combination of dopamine- and acetylcholine-boosting medications. He's been at his most recent job for over six months—a record for Tom—and he's taking night classes to get his high school diploma.

Attention deficit disorder and attention deficit hyperactivity disorder (which are also sometimes called hyperkinetic disorder) affect 3 to 9 percent of children in the United States—about four times more boys than girls. The kids who have it tend to be smart, but they have trouble focusing, become bored and frustrated easily, and they are frequently in motion—running, jumping, swinging—but they are also often awkward and uncoordinated. They tend to act out a lot and have trouble following directions. Perhaps as a result of some of those problems, they often do poorly in school, suffer from low-self esteem, and have problems interacting with their peers. Although we rarely hear about it, kids are not the only ones with ADD and ADHD. In fact, there are 8 to 12 million adults with ADD or ADHD.

What does this have to do with warming deficits? If a deficit of heat and motivation reduces activity, you might be wondering how it could possibly cause ADD and ADHD, which are conditions commonly associated with hyperactivity. Here's how it works: the brain has a built-in filtration system that enables you to ignore everything extraneous to what you're doing. That's why you can carry on a conversation with one person in a restaurant and not be incredibly distracted by what's going on at all the other tables. Basically, the filter is an inhibitor that allows you to focus on one thing at a time. When there isn't enough dopamine, the filter doesn't work as well, and it becomes difficult or impossible to focus on anything for any more than a few minutes. Dopamine stimulates this filter, which then allows you to ignore other distractions.

Another view of the connection between ADD and neurotransmitters places some of the blame on acetylcholine deficiency. Even though acetylcholine is a warming neurotransmitter, part of its function is to stimulate the mechanisms that *stop* things. Without enough acetylcholine to balance things out, the sympathetic nervous system can get out of control, resulting in frenetic activity. Stimulants trigger an increase in dopamine as well as a smaller increase in acetylcholine, which makes dopamine even more effective. Researchers are currently looking at acetylcholine-enhancing drugs because of their effect on enhancing attention span, though they tend not to work as well as dopamine-enhancing drugs.

One fascinating theory is that ADD and ADHD are actually reward deficiency conditions, similar in a way to addictive behavior. Think about it this way. There are two ways to learn: positive reinforcement (giving pleasure) and negative reinforcement (giving pain). When something happens that isn't associated with some degree of pleasure or pain, our brain hardly takes notice. By releasing dopamine, ADD and ADHD drugs are giving some significance to things that previously would have gone unnoticed (such as the need to sit down, focus, or respond to discipline), and telling the brain that those things are worth paying attention to.

That's the positive reinforcement method. The negative reinforcement method—which would involve glutamate-enhancing drugs—doesn't really exist, and there's a good reason why. We know that the higher the levels of glutamate in the brain, the more pain we can perceive. The problem is that excessive amounts of glutamate are responsible for brain damage and a number of degenerative conditions.

SAD and Warming Deficiency

Keesha was a forty-four-year-old owner of a food and beverage company that supplies items to major theme parks and sports stadiums. She came to see Chris late one December, complaining of "feeling down, just not feeling myself" for several months. She had just returned from having spent the holidays with her brother and her family and had barely made it through the week.

Keesha said that there were many times when she had to leave the room because she felt she would begin crying at any moment. She slept ten hours a night but woke up feeling tired and as if her head was in a fog. She ate candy and drank coffee nonstop but got no boost.

Keesha felt guilty about having symptoms of what she thought was depression—her business was doing well, her family members were all healthy, and she didn't have a reason in the world to feel depressed. The day before Keesha left, her brother took her aside and asked what was wrong. At the suggestion that she might be having trouble, Keesha broke into tears and told her brother that she had no idea what was bothering her.

Keesha's brother had a possible answer. He reminded Keesha that their mother used to get depressed every winter when they were growing up in Chicago. He added that he'd had the same kinds of symptoms for several years, until he finally went to see his doctor, who diagnosed him with seasonal affective disorder (SAD). He tried several medications before settling on Elavil. He offered Keesha a few of his pills, but Keesha wisely declined.

During their initial consultation, Chris found out that Keesha spent the majority of her time indoors during the winter, rarely getting out until spring. She also drank more beer in the winter than during the summer. Both of these behaviors created a warming neurotransmitter deficiency. Chris suggested Wellbutrin, but Keesha said she preferred to try a nonprescription treatment. Chris had Keesha buy Ott lamps for her home and office and suggested that she replace the fluorescent light bulbs at work with full-spectrum bulbs to increase the intensity of light her brain received each day. He also told Keesha to abstain from beer and other alcohol and spend at least twenty minutes outside every day. After a week, he put her on the Warming Program described in this book.

A month later, when Keesha came back for her follow-up appointment, she said she was "100 percent better," and was no longer tired or depressed. Her energy level was so much improved that she started working out in a gym. "That," she said, "really made a difference."

Have you ever felt a little sluggish, sad, unmotivated, a little depressed, or just plain blah in the late fall or winter? If those symptoms lasted only a few days, all you've got is a mild case of the winter blues. But if those symptoms last for longer than a few days or if they become oppressive or even debilitating, you may be one of the estimated 10 to 15 million Americans (75 to 80 percent of whom are women) who suffer from seasonal affective disorder. SAD is a real disorder with severe, sometimes life-threatening consequences.

No one is sure what causes SAD or why some people get it and others don't. But some of the evidence points to a group of about 10,000 neurons called the *suprachiasmatic nucleus* (SCN), which is generally accepted as being our internal master clock, the thing that synchronizes all of the rhythms that keep us alive, from sleeping and waking to breathing and heart rate. The SCN regulates these cycles in part based on the amount of light it receives (it's actually located just above the *optic chaisma,* which is right behind the eyes).

Several studies indicate that low levels of light are associated with lower dopamine production in the brain. This fact fits perfectly with our binary model, in which warming NTs such as dopamine are dominant in the daytime, while the cooling NTs are dominant at night. SAD is also more common in northern geographical areas or areas that get less light in the winter. Symptoms can include any or all of the following:

- weight gain
- drop in energy level
- fatigue
- sad or empty feeling
- loss of interest in things that used to be pleasurable
- difficulty concentrating
- irritability
- tendency to oversleep or not want to get out of bed
- craving for sugary or starchy foods

Symptoms generally start in the fall or winter and disappear by May or so. There is also a much rarer summer variation, whose symptoms can include depression, poor appetite, weight loss, and insomnia.

Chronic Fatigue and Warming Deficiency

Dopamine is all about creation and destruction and is responsible for movement, energy, and motivation. By moving molecules and us into action, it destroys the status quo, which is maintained by serotonin. Researchers at Johns Hopkins University have linked low levels of dopamine and norepinephrine with many of the symptoms most commonly associated with chronic fatigue syndrome—nearly constant exhaustion and foggy thinking. Low dopamine and/or norepinephrine levels interfere with adequate blood flow to the brain, which then causes fatigue. Researchers call this *neurally mediated hypotension.*

PMS and Warming Deficiency

Premenstrual syndrome (PMS) affects an estimated 25 million women, typically between ovulation and the start of menstruation. Although people have a tendency to talk about PMS as if it were a single condition, there are over 150 different symptoms, ranging from anxiety, cramps, and mood swings to forgetfulness, insomnia, swelling, and tenderness. As you might expect, different symptoms are associated with different neurotransmitter imbalances. The ones specifically associated with warming NT deficiencies include:

- depression
- bloating
- breast swelling and tenderness
- morning face puffiness

Karen's Story:
Warming Deficiency and PMS

Chris had a patient, Karen, who came to see him hoping for some relief from her PMS-related symptoms: breast swelling and tenderness, tearfulness, and extreme fatigue. Karen, a thirty-five-year-old caterer, was big boned, 10 to 20 pounds overweight but not obese, and she looked worn down. Still, she spoke clearly, stating her intentions, concerns, and desires in a steady, engaging way.

Karen worked long hours and told Chris that she always worried about being able to keep up the pace. She felt as though the world was moving too fast and demanding too much from her. As a result, she didn't eat well. "I'm always on the run," she said. "I never eat, I just pick and nibble." She didn't sleep well either, getting only five and a half to six and a half hours a night. Not surprisingly, she was too tired to do any regular exercise.

Karen's lack of energy and constant attempts to keep up had depleted her warming neurotransmitters. To raise those levels, Chris began by putting Karen on the 28-day program described on pages 131–179. He also had Karen listen to rhythmic music, which stimulates dopamine production, in her car and at work.

After a month, Karen felt much better—more energetic and less frazzled. Her PMS symptoms were also greatly reduced. But she wanted more. Chris suggested that she stay on the diet, but added small amounts of three herbs that have been shown to increase warming neurotransmitters. Again, after a few weeks there was even more improvement, but Karen still wasn't feeling as good as she thought she could.

Chris then ordered some tests and found that Karen's hormone levels were out of balance—particularly her estrogen level, which was too high. Since estrogen is a cooling hormone (as opposed to testosterone, which is warming), this was clearly adding to her warming deficiency. As it happened, Karen's birth control pills turned out to be the culprit. Changing to a different method restored Karen's hormone levels to normal and completely resolved her PMS symptoms.

Menopause and Warming Deficiency

For women, simply being postmenopausal is a risk factor for a deficiency of acetylcholine, which influences the body's estrogen levels. This is why many women experiencing PMS and menopause feel they are losing their ability to think and remember. In reality, they're undergoing a temporary but potentially permanent loss of cognitive function.

Preserving cognitive ability during menopause requires more than estrogen replacement therapy. The solution involves a comprehensive approach directed at balancing brain chemistry. Treating menopause from its earliest recognizable stages using diet, exercise, sleep, and perspective forms a foundation of support that minimizes the deleterious effects of the declining reproductive hormones. Supporting neurotransmitter activity maintains order during an otherwise chaotic period in a woman's personal evolution and development. Comprehensive hormone replacement, customized to address each perimenopausal woman's needs, assists the brain in its ability to perform the complex functions that underlie health and vitality.

Male Menopause and Warming Deficiency

As men's testosterone levels decline in midlife, men experience many of the same emotional traumas—particularly depression—that women experience as their estrogen levels drop. Testosterone closely parallels dopamine, and decreasing levels are associated with many dopamine-deficit conditions, including depression, reduced libido, erectile or sexual dysfunction, fatigue, confusion, and a number of declines in cognitive performance. Men who take testosterone report that they have an increased sex drive, feel more aggressive in business transactions, and are less irritable, happier, and generally more content. The signs and symptoms of male menopause are far more variable and inconsistent than those of female menopause. But that doesn't make them any less serious. (It's interesting to note that blood testosterone levels fluctuate throughout the day, peaking at 8:00 A.M.—just about the time that dopamine levels peak—and dropping to their lowest levels at about 8:00 P.M.—just when the cooling neurotransmitters take over.)

Aging and Warming Deficiency

As we get older, our neurotransmitter receptors become less sensitive, which effectively reduces the amount of NTs that the body and brain can make use of. The result is a series of gradual changes that we typically associate with aging, such as loss of body mass, reduced energy and motivation, balance difficulties, memory loss, increased risk of mood disorders, and decreased cardiac function. All of these conditions are linked to deficits of dopamine, acetylcholine, and norepinephrine. When warming neurotransmitter levels are low, the body's ability to regenerate and repair itself is impaired.

Research has shown a clear connection between advancing age and increased *monoamine oxidase* (MAO), which is the enzyme that degrades both dopamine and serotonin. As we age, levels of both of these vital neurotransmitters fall, leaving us increasingly vulnerable to depression, dementia, Parkinson's, and orthostatic blood pressure changes (how your blood pressure changes as you move from sitting or lying to standing or sitting).

In addition, dopamine plays a role in overall cognitive ability. A team of researchers at the National Institutes of Aging recently completed a study of men aged fifty-one to ninety-one. They followed the men for ten years, tracking their blood testosterone levels and their performance on a number of cognitive tests, including verbal and visual memory, visuomotor scanning and attention, verbal knowledge, and spatial ability. The researchers found that declining levels of testosterone (which parallel brain dopamine levels) were associated with losses in overall cognitive performance. Conversely, the higher the testosterone levels, the better the overall cognitive performance. We'll talk about the advantages and disadvantages of testosterone replacement for both men and women on pages 181–182.

Your Heart and Warming Deficiency

Our bodies—and every organ and system within them—are essentially binary, meaning they have two states: on (warmed or excited) and off (cooled or inhibited). The same is true of your *autonomic nervous system,* which is better known as the "fight-or-flight response." The on and off parts of the autonomic nervous system are the *sympathetic* and the *parasympathetic.*

The sympathetic system is essentially your body's 911 emergency alert system. It's predominantly governed by norepinephrine, and your heart is right at the center of it. If you have been mugged or have experienced any scary or life-threatening situation, you know exactly how this feels: your heart rate and blood pressure increase, your blood vessels constrict, you sweat, your muscles contract, your mind goes into a state of super-awareness, and you're ready for anything.

When dopamine and norepinephrine levels are in proper balance, your heart beats regularly and rhythmically and adjusts the amount of blood it pumps to whatever situation you happen to be in. An excess of these neurotransmitters puts you into a sympathetic state too often for no real reason. One example of this is panic disorder, which is what happens when the brain's alarm system is continually and inappropriately activated by norepinephrine.

A deficiency has the opposite effect, making it impossible for you to initiate a sympathetic response when you really need it. Without enough dopamine and norepinephrine your cardiovascular function is impaired and your heart gradually loses its ability to respond appropriately. (If you were mugged, for example, your heart rate and blood pressure might not change at all.) Your pulse slows and your blood pressure drops, and the heart's pumping capacity is reduced. You get dizzy when you stand up or change position, and as your circulation slows, further swelling occurs, especially in the feet and ankles.

Ultimately, the low blood pressure and slow pulse can result in congestive heart failure. A standard emergency room treatment for acute heart failure is an IV of dopamine.

Pain and Warming Deficiency

It makes sense that since dopamine is an essential agent of pleasure and reward, a dopamine deficiency would cause discomfort. When we are dopamine deficient, we feel a variety of pains and annoyances that we call hunger, thirst, lust, depression, and cravings for foods, drugs, or other dopamine-increasing substances. Buddhists say that "all desire is pain," and dopamine is the neurotransmitter of desire. Pain is essential for survival. Without it we wouldn't be able to stop doing dangerous things or get out of threatening situations. It would be much more difficult to learn and nearly impossible to change. Once recognized, the pain of dopamine deficiency can be used in its earliest stages to motivate us toward the behaviors, environments, foods, vitamins, and other agents known to stimulate dopamine and restore balance.

Addictions and Cravings and Warming Deficiency

Our brain comes fully equipped with its very own pleasure and reward centers, areas that, when stimulated, release dopamine, which, in turn, produces feelings of pleasure. These "natural rewards" are what motivate us to engage in the two activities most essential to our survival: eating and reproducing. One of these pleasure centers was discovered by accident in 1954 by the psychologist James Olds, who was studying the "state of alertness" in rats. Olds mistakenly placed some electrodes deeper into the brain than he had intended and touched a cluster of cells called the *nucleus accumbens*. When the rats' brains were wired so they could give themselves a jolt of dopamine by pressing a lever that stimulated the nucleus accumbens, Olds found that the animals did so nearly nonstop, as many as 5,000 times an hour, enduring any adversity and forgetting about eating, drinking, sleeping, or sex until they pleasured themselves to death. Olds had found the ultimate in self-stimulation and reward.

Research on human subjects has revealed that in addition to the nucleus accumbens, there are pleasure centers in the *locus coerleus* and the *globus pallidus*. When stimulated, these centers release and activate dopamine neurons, which produce feelings ranging from ecstasy to the obliteration of all negative thought.

A number of substances such as cocaine, amphetamines, cigarettes, heroin, nicotine, caffeine, and compulsive behavior such as gambling, sex, and adrenaline thrills also stimulate these pleasure centers and trigger the same dopamine release and the corresponding feelings of pleasure. These are called "unnatural rewards." The big problem with unnatural rewards is that the surge of dopamine you get from addictive drugs is far greater than what you get when you eat or have sex or engage in one of the more traditional pleasure-enhancing activities. As a result, the brain decides that whatever just triggered the dopamine release is the best thing that's ever happened to it, and will do almost anything to feel that way again.

Drug and alcohol use also causes permanent physiological changes in the brain. The first thing that happens is that the brain develops a tolerance, meaning that it takes more and more of whatever stimulated it to make it happy. After a while, the addict or alcoholic needs some kind of unnatural reward just to get to the point of feeling "normal." If he doesn't get what he needs, he starts going through withdrawal, which can be very painful—both physically and emotionally.

Although many typically see addiction of all kinds as a type of character flaw, the truth is that addiction is a disease akin to diabetes or lupus. Some people are born with an abnormally low density of dopamine receptors in the nucleus accumbens. This deficit reduces the individual's ability to experience pleasure, so he or she will crave substances that offer some kind of relief from the deficiency. There's some indication that this type of dopamine deficiency is hereditary. Adopted children whose biological parents were alcoholics are far more likely to become alcoholics themselves than children whose biological parents aren't alcoholic.

Other people develop a dopamine deficiency because of the way they're raised or the environment they live in. Children who are physically or emotionally mistreated, who are repeatedly told they're worthless (or stupid or will never amount to anything), or who grow up deprived of the most basic needs produce less dopamine. As a result, they may end up looking to artificial means to restore balance.

You don't have to have substance abusing parents or grow up in a dysfunctional family to develop a dopamine deficiency. Although certain people are certainly predisposed toward addictive behavior, even those whose dopamine levels start off perfectly normal can get into bad habits. If a dopamine deficiency isn't there already, repeated alcohol or drug use can create one.

Addictive behavior seems to be a combination of a deficit of pain sensitivity (which would otherwise keep someone from doing stupid or self-destructive things), a deficit of pleasure (which continually motivates the person to seek pleasure), and the *threat* of the pain that would come from not giving in to the craving for the drugs. It's that threat alone that accounts for the fact that about three quarters of those who go through drug rehab programs relapse within six months.

Although dopamine is considered to be the neurotransmitter most involved in addiction, recent research indicates that glutamate may play an equally important role. Scientists at the University of California –San Francisco and Stanford noticed that cocaine triggers a change in glutamate activity that is remarkably similar to the changes that happen during long-term potentiation (the mechanism the brain uses to create long-term memories). This may explain why it's so easy for former drug addicts to relapse, even after years on the wagon. These changes are so powerful to a former addict that often just seeing drug paraphernalia or being in a place where he used to do drugs can be enough to spark cravings and, possibly, relapse, according to a recent article in *Nature*. In experiments with rats, the researchers were able to prevent relapse by giving them a glutamate-blocking drug.

Cigarettes.   Nicotine has an effect on three neurotransmitters. It raises serotonin, which gives the smoker a feeling of being full and reduces the appetite. When the smoker quits, serotonin levels return to normal and the appetite returns. This explains why so many people gain weight after they stop smoking. But it's nicotine's ability to increase dopamine and norepinephrine (both warming NTs) in the pleasure centers of the brain that causes the actual addiction. Cigarettes are often people's first experience with addiction, and nicotine seems to pave the way for other addictions.

Caffeine.   By raising serotonin levels, caffeine gives the coffee drinker a warm, safe feeling. But it also significantly increases dopamine, which provides that buzz that so many people depend on to get through their day.

Cocaine.   Cocaine increases serotonin and dopamine. But because it also blocks dopamine reuptake (reabsorption), more dopamine stays in the system. When that dopamine finally goes away, the need to restore it to artificially high levels is overwhelming. That's what addiction is all about.

Food Cravings, Obesity, and Warming Deficiency

Neurotransmitters have a direct effect on our appetite and food preferences and on how we regulate our nutrient balance. The word *calorie* means "to heat" or "to burn." And since dopamine is our principal warming neurotransmitter, it shouldn't come as much of a surprise that it's involved in burning calories. At the same time, since serotonin is about cooling, it's natural that its job would be to conserve energy by slowing down the rate at which calories are burned.

Food cravings, especially for sweet and starchy foods, are just like an addiction. Those kinds of foods break down in our bloodstream, change our mood, and make us feel better (temporarily). The more you give in, the more dependent you'll become and the harder it will be to break the addiction. Even the *anticipation* of the dopamine-induced pleasure that food will produce triggers the desire to eat as well as a slight increase in dopamine. That quickly breaks down into norepinephrine, which makes you physically move—lifting your fork, opening the refrigerator, or whatever. As soon as you take a bite, you get the dopamine you were looking for, immediately followed by a small burst of serotonin that slows you down. Since dopamine is metabolized much faster than serotonin, after a while you end up with a relative surplus of serotonin, which makes you full.

Stress creates a state of imbalance in which action and inflammation predominate. Together, the warming NTs and their allies keep sugar in the blood, halt cell repair and maintenance activities, and shift us into fight-or-flight mode. If the triggers of acute stress are pulled daily or if the alarm or sense of threat is never completely damped, our appetites change along with our senses of taste and smell, how our bodies respond to food, and ultimately how we look and feel. The adaptive steps the brain and body take in order to cope with chronic stress often lead to the urges, actions, and responses that contribute to obesity.

If you're a warming deficient person, your brain may want more pleasure-inducing foods even though you're not really hungry anymore—the classic definition of overeating. The potential dopamine reward is too tempting to pass by. So the brain triggers a craving for that extra piece of pizza, another beer, a third piece of cake, some chocolate, or any other rich, sugary, or fatty food. (Few people overeat foods that trigger a cooling response such as diet crackers or vegetables.) Since we all have occasional warming neurotransmitter deficiencies, this kind of thing happens to everyone once in a while. But if the warming deficiency is severe enough or lasts long enough, it can lead to obesity.

Dr. Kishore Gadde and his colleagues at Duke University put fifty nondepressed overweight and obese women on a 1,600-calorie-per-day diet. He also gave them the dopamine-enhancing drug Wellbutrin.

After only eight weeks, 67 percent of the women had lost an average of 5 percent of their body weight (compared to only 15 percent of the women on the same diet but taking a placebo instead of Wellbutrin). Ordinarily, low-cal diets result in loss of lean muscle tissue, plus there's the risk of lost bone density and osteoporosis. But the women in the Wellbutrin group in this study lost most of their weight in fat. And after a total of 24 weeks on the diet, they showed no loss of bone density.

Diabetes and Insulin Resistance and Warming Deficiency

Brain cells use glucose as an energy source, but eating a high-carbohydrate (or high-sugar) diet raises insulin levels, which basically floods the cells with sugar. As a kind of defense mechanism, your cells develop *insulin resistance,* which makes them less responsive to insulin. The less responsive your cells are to insulin, the less sensitized they are to dopamine, which is why eating a lot of carbohydrates can leave you feeling sluggish and tired (after the initial boost you sometimes get). If this situation continues, you'll develop *insulin resistance syndrome,* otherwise known as *Syndrome X,* a condition whose symptoms are a combination of elevated LDL (bad) cholesterol, blood pressure, blood sugar, insulin, low HDL (good) cholesterol, and obesity (in the form of an apple-shaped body).

Low dopamine carries other risks as well. Patients who use dopamine-blocking drugs have a five times greater risk of developing diabetes than patients who don't.

Sex and Warming Deficiency

There's very little argument with the theory that dopamine has a major influence over our sex lives. As already noted, dopamine is the neurotransmitter that regulates our ability to perceive and experience pleasure. And what could be more pleasurable than sex? Dopamine excites, pursues, and conquers. It increases sensory perception and heightens awareness. Acetylcholine gets our sex organs ready for action.

Studies have shown that dopamine production increases during foreplay. There's also a large, sustained increase in dopamine in the *nucleus accumbens* (one of the brain's pleasure centers) during sexual activity. This increase drops off sharply after ejaculation or orgasm, as our cooling NTs kick in.

In animal studies, dopamine-blocking drugs reduce rates of sexual behavior in male rats. And as we discuss in chapter 4, many serotonin-enhancing drugs (often called selective serotonin reuptake inhibitors or SSRI) reduce the libido. One of the ways doctors have of countering that undesirable side effect is to augment the SSRI with a dopamine-enhancing drug such as Wellbutrin (see page 183).

Our other warming NTs are involved too. While dopamine offers small rewards for pursuing a partner, norepinephrine helps us focus, glutamate helps us learn the ins and outs of mating and sexual behavior, and acetylcholine heightens sensory sensitivity and prepares our sexual organs. Acetylcholine also mediates the release of *pheromones,* the invisible chemicals of sexual perception that purportedly help us choose among potential sex partners.

Your Bones and Warming Deficiency

Two recent discoveries highlight the connection between dopamine and your bones. We now know that bones contain dopamine receptors, and we know that the gene for bone development is remarkably similar to the one for dopamine synthesis. Both of these discoveries highlight the interesting connection between dopamine and the strength and growth of your skeletal structure. People who are on dopamine-blocking drugs, for example, frequently have less dense and more fragile bones than those who are not.

In addition, drugs that block dopamine cause the pituitary gland to secrete prolactin. Excessive amounts of prolactin have been linked with a drop in estrogen levels, which is a known risk factor for osteoporosis in women.

Sleep and Warming Deficiency

Sleep is absolutely critical to our survival. One of its major functions was especially important back in our caveman days, when the urge to sleep was actually a protective measure, designed to keep us out of circulation when predators—whose sense of smell, hearing, and night vision are far better than our own—were about. Today, sleep's restorative functions—the time it gives our brain and body to rest and repair themselves—are far more important.

Experts used to believe that your brain was more active when you're awake, and that activity drops when you're asleep. Now we know that wakefulness and sleep states are equally active—they're just controlled by different parts of the brain. Cooling NTs are more active at night, while warming NTs are more active during the day. A cooling deficit causes a relative excess of warming, which would lead to insomnia or difficulty staying asleep. On the other hand, a warming deficit causes the opposite situation—a relative excess of cooling and excessive sleep.

Different warming deficits affect our sleep in different ways. Do you have problems recalling your dreams? That's probably a lack of acetylcholine. Acetylcholine agonists have been shown to increase dreaming and trigger a process known as *shortened REM latency* (meaning that dreams come quicker).

Interestingly, despite the allure of sleeping in, it turns out that too much sleep may be even worse for you than too little. Daniel Gottlieb of the Boston University School of Medicine analyzed fourteen years' worth of data on over 4,500 men and women and found that people who slept for nine hours or longer were 70 percent more likely to die than those who slept seven to eight hours. Those who slept six hours or less had a 50 percent greater chance of dying than the seven-to-eight-hour group.

Parkinson's Disease and Warming Deficiency

Parkinson's is primarily a disease of the motor system. The major marker is progressive loss of dopamine-manufacturing neurons in the *substantia nigra* of the brain. Symptoms include tremors, rigidity, and severe limitations of movement. Parkinson's patients also commonly develop "secondary" dopamine deficiency–related symptoms such as depression, senility, postural deformity, difficulty in speaking, and even dementia in the disease's late stages.

If you have *any* of these symptoms, see your doctor immediately. Parkinson's is a progressive, degenerative disease, whose early symptoms are minor enough that many people have no idea that they are affected.

Certain dopamine-depleting drugs may induce Parkinson's-like symptoms after as little as one dose. These include Haldol (an antipsychotic) and several drugs for nausea and vomiting such as Compazine and Reglan. These Parkinson's-like symptoms can be reversed, but Parkinson's cannot. Used for a long period of time, these drugs may actually cause Parkinson's. On the other hand, boosting dopamine levels with dopamine-stimulating drugs dramatically reduces the symptoms. (Dopamine-stimulating drugs also reduce the symptoms of depression that commonly accompany Parkinson's.)

The irony of using dopamine-stimulating drugs, such as the dopamine precursor levodopa, is that they improve movement for a while (a period called the *Parkinson holiday*) but then lose their effect, leaving the Parkinson's patient in a progressive downhill decline. No one is sure why this happens, but one interesting theory has it that Parkinson's is actually preceded by an excess of dopamine (too much warming), which stimulates more activity than the brain can safely handle. This dopamine overload makes the brain produce a lot of energy but also creates waste and cell damage from chemical reactions that give off *free radicals.* The suspicion is that this damage triggers a shutdown of the *substantia nigra,* the area of the brain where dopamine is produced. This, in turn, causes the dopamine deficiency that leads to Parkinson's.

Replacing or stimulating dopamine production without addressing the patients' inability to protect themselves from excessive dopamine activity ultimately destroys the few remaining dopamine-producing cells and causes the precipitous and irreversible decline in their condition. Several researchers studying new Parkinson's treatments have found augmenting dopamine-stimulating drugs with melatonin (a serotonin by-product) can protect the patient and extend levodopa's benefits.

Cancer and Warming Deficiency

The link between neurotransmitters and cancer goes back several thousand years. In about 400 B.C., Hippocrates believed that cancer—breast cancer in particular—was the result of an imbalance of one of the four humors. About five hundred years later, Galen, a Greek physician, claimed that melancholia (depression) was the chief cause of breast cancer. Fifteen hundred years later still, direct connections are being made.

In 2002, Philip Wang, a researcher in the Division of Pharmacoepidemiology and Pharmacoeconomics at Brigham and Women's Hospital, completed a study of over 100,000 women. Half were taking dopamine antagonists (blocking drugs), the other half were not. Over a period of about six and a half years, Wang found that the women who were taking the dopamine blockers had a 16 percent higher risk of breast cancer.

Cancer and Stress

Under normal circumstances, levels of the stress hormone cortisol vary throughout the day: higher in the morning, lower at night. (Since cortisol is a warming hormone, it makes sense that it would be more active in the morning, when the warming neurotransmitters are dominant, and less active in the evening, when the cooling neurotransmitters are dominant.) Some women with advanced breast cancer, however, have abnormal cortisol levels, sometimes remaining flat throughout the day or peaking at the wrong times, according to David Spiegel, a researcher at Stanford University medical school. Patients who had these patterns died much earlier than patients whose patterns were normal.

Cortisol is a natural immune system suppressant, and patients with abnormal cortisol patterns also had depressed levels of cells that kill cancer cells. In addition, Spiegel points out that cortisol sends signals that cause normal cells to release glucose into the blood, but cancerous cells don't respond to those signals. As a result, cancer cells have more glucose to use for energy and are able to resist an already weakened immune system.

Cancer and Depression

William Eaton and his colleagues at the Johns Hopkins School of Public Health found that women with a history of depression were four times more likely to develop breast cancer than those who had never been clinically depressed. The same team is currently investigating whether there's a similar link between prostate cancer and depression, since both breast and prostate cancers are hormonally related. Depression doesn't seem to be a major risk factor for other types of cancer.

Harry's Story: Warming Deficiencies, Cancer, and Depression

In a sense, Harry, a fifty-six-year-old retired businessman, lived like most Americans. He didn't exercise at all, and he ate a diet that was extremely high in saturated fats and sugars. That combination undoubtedly explained why he was 20 percent overweight. He woke up earlier than he wanted to but couldn't get back to sleep. He was taking several medications to deal with heart and cholesterol problems, and he was extremely depressed because he had prostate cancer that had metastasized to the bone.

Chris did several tests and confirmed that Harry had low levels of testosterone (due to his prostate cancer treatment), thyroid, and growth hormone.

Chris also did some allergy testing and put Harry on an anti-inflammatory diet to deal with the weight issue, had him promise to start exercising regularly to improve his mood, and prescribed Sonata as a way to get back to sleep. He augmented Harry's nutrition program with a number of nutritional supplements but could not boost his testosterone, thyroid, growth hormone, or DHEA levels due to the possible link between these hormones and cancer growth. He did, however, prescribe DHEA-K, a form of DHEA that does not convert into testosterone yet still supports warming NT function. Chris designed this program specifically to increase Harry's warming neurotransmitters. In order to avoid stimulating the prostate cancer and metastasis, he deliberately avoided anything that would increase his testosterone or growth hormone.

Under the guidance of his oncologist, Harry did a course of chemotherapy. He's been in remission for eleven months, and he credits Chris's program with helping him stay strong through the chemo and for reducing his PSA from 28 to 3.

As someone with a warming deficiency, you're a little too cool for your own good. You're more sedentary than you should be, and you eat more starchy foods and sleep a little longer than you probably should. Plus, you're a little less optimistic and excited and a little more depressed than is comfortable. All of these traits create their own unique challenges in your daily life, the biggest being that they make you vulnerable to the symptoms and diseases we've discussed in this chapter. In chapter 6, you'll find a 28-day plan that contains the tools you need to heal yourself and restore the balance that's just right for you. The results will amaze you: you'll feel more energetic and less depressed; you'll be able to think more clearly and your memory and ability to concentrate will improve; chronic conditions you may be suffering from will get better, and you'll feel more healthy, fit, and attractive.

CHAPTER 4

Are You Too Warm?

How Cooling Deficiencies Affect Your Mind and Body

One of Chris's patients is Britt, a forty-five-year-old documentary filmmaker who has traveled the world, creating award-winning films on every subject from the extinction of indigenous creatures to cooperation among the nations working on the international space station.

Britt came in with a number of symptoms that indicated a cooling deficiency: irritability, loss of concentration, inability to sleep without frequent awakening, urinary urgency, and periods of fatigue that were interfering with his work. He also had a chronic sore throat and recurring symptoms of sinusitis that seemed to get worse every time he worked in Los Angeles or almost anywhere else. Before seeing Chris, Britt had consulted with three other doctors. The first one diagnosed Britt as being "allergic to everything" and suggested that he create a hypoallergenic environment in his multiple homes, which he did. The doctor also prescribed allergy shots that worked for a while but then wore off, leaving Britt as allergic as ever.

The second doctor ordered tests, which came back normal. He diagnosed Britt as suffering from sinusitis and prescribed antibiotics. Again, Britt complied with the doctor's orders, but by the time he completed his course of antibiotics he was feeling worse than ever.

Britt was about to embark on a costly three-month project in a remote location abroad and was worried that he wouldn't be able to make it. The third doctor prescribed more antibiotics and added some sleeping pills. The first prescription he received was too weak and did not help him sleep; the second was too strong and left him feeling drowsy the next day.

Britt arrived in Chris's office two days before he was due to leave. He said he was desperate for help but was planning to go forward with the project despite his health concerns. Chris explained the concept of neurotransmitter imbalances and cooling deficiencies in particular and suggested trying to reduce Britt's inflammation over the long term by correcting his cooling neurotransmitter deficiency.

Chris put Britt on a 28-day program very much like the one in chapter 7. The first step was some basic mental techniques designed to help Britt deal with his stress by adjusting his thoughts and feelings. Chris gave Britt instructions to do stretching exercises every day as a way to gently stimulate his cooling neurotransmitters, and he gave him a natural sleep aid, 5-HTP. The next step would have been to send Britt out for comprehensive food allergy testing. But because Britt was leaving the country, Chris suggested that he eliminate sugar and caffeine and avoid eating the most common allergenic foods (wheat, dairy, eggs, soy, and peanuts). He also recommended a three-day rotation diet, eating foods no more frequently than three days apart in order to avoid developing additional food sensitivities.

Three days later, Britt called Chris to tell him how much better he felt after implementing the relaxation techniques, doing the exercises, and following the diet. His sore throat and sinus symptoms were gone. After eliminating the offending foods, Britt noticed that he no longer had to clear his throat repeatedly during his meals, and that he felt more energetic more of the time.

The relationship between his symptoms and his diet and tension had become immediately apparent. After two weeks he e-mailed that he was sleeping through the night with only an occasional awakening and his urinary urgency had resolved. He felt his concentration was back and he no longer had flares of irritability. After twenty-eight days he felt so much better that he continued the diet and the physical and mental exercises and no longer needed the natural sleep aids.

Britt sent Chris a copy of the finished documentary and looked stronger and more vital than ever. He had not only helped himself regain his balance but also learned a series of techniques he can use over and over again any time he feels the symptoms of cooling deficiency.

When was the last time you felt truly satisfied and content, completely at peace, and confident that all was right with the world? It's probably been quite a while—and even when you had that wonderful feeling, we're sure it didn't last as long as you wanted it to. What you experience on the rare occasions when you feel this way is what it's like when you have adequate levels of cooling neurotransmitters in your brain. The rest of the time—which is most of the time—those cooling neurotransmitters, serotonin and GABA, are out of balance and life isn't nearly as pleasant as it could be. You may have an imbalance of serotonin and GABA, your major cooling neurotransmitters. Symptoms of this kind of imbalance may include:

- always feeling anxious or on edge
- restlessness and insomnia or lethargy and fatigue
- tight or twitching muscles
- eating disorders or irritable bowel syndrome
- shortness of breath
- migraines
- darkness under the eyes
- depression
- angry outbursts
- obsessive or compulsive behavior
- nausea

At first glance, a lot of the symptoms we'll describe in this chapter—such as anger and impulsiveness—will seem more related to heat than to cooling. There's a reason for that. In chapter 1 we talked about the connections between ancient systems of medicine and our current understanding of neurochemistry. A traditional Chinese healer, for example, would say that someone exhibiting the symptoms in this chapter is suffering from a deficit of water. We'd say that person has a deficit of cooling neurotransmitters—or an excess of heating ones—and we'd use metaphors like being hot under the collar, being a hothead, having a temper that boils over, burning the candle at both ends, needing to cool off or "chill," being consumed with passion, and so on.

When it comes to brain chemistry, heat is more than a metaphor. Stress and anger raise body temperature, and relaxation lowers it. If the brain can't provide enough cooling influence to balance out the heat, a temperature increase that goes too high or lasts too long can cause delusions, mania, heart attacks, and even serious brain damage. What the overheated or undercooled patient needs to regain control is to throw a little water on the fire. And that's what serotonin and GABA, our major cooling neurotransmitters, do for us—they reduce the activity of dopamine and the other heating neurotransmitters.

That raises an interesting question: Are cooling deficits really cooling deficits or are they actually an excess of heat? The answer is yes and yes. When serotonin is deficient, the heating effects of dopamine and glutamate overstimulate the brain. In a sense, an excess of heat is, by definition, a deficiency of cool, and vice versa. Some of the symptoms you'll read about in this chapter are specifically caused by abnormally low levels of cooling NTs; others by abnormally high heat levels. In both cases, most of the time the symptoms can be resolved by increasing serotonin. Some cases, however, require blocking dopamine and/or glutamate.

Our cooling NTs play a role in nearly every aspect of our lives—every decision we make, every pleasure we feel, and every act great or small. They keep us from overreacting and allow us to feel pleasure. When we're scared, they comfort us; when we're hot, they cool us; and when we're nervous, they calm us. When stress, pressure, anger, and the lack of desire or motivation make life almost intolerable, our cooling NTs make it better. Together, they influence our:

* emotions, mood, and feelings of security
* energy level and motivation
* sexual desires
* critical brain functions, including speed of thought and ability to acquire new information
* digestive function
* weight
* ability to enjoy life

Let's take a look at where our cooling NTs come from and some of the ways they work—independently and together—to affect our minds, emotions, bodies, and behavior.

Serotonin

Serotonin is produced from the amino acid L-tryptophan in an area of the brain called the *raphe nuclei,* which is located in the brain stem at the very top of the spine. The raphe nuclei uses an intricate web of pathways to send serotonin to over a dozen receptors in other areas of the brain, including those that control our cardiovascular (heart) and thermoregulatory (temperature regulation) systems. The most important serotonin receptor is in the *hypothalamus,* the small but critical part of the brain that manages everything related to the survival of the species, what some people call the "four Fs": feeding, fighting, fleeing, and, well, having sex.

When our serotonin levels are balanced we feel safe and fulfilled. Too little and we become hypervigilant, worry about the unknown, and begin to doubt ourselves, and our body's ability to defend itself against hostile microbes diminishes. Too much and our systems slow down. We can get fat, lose our motivation and our desire to have sex, and become lazy and sedentary. Serotonin is probably the most important NT when it comes to maintaining good mood and a positive outlook on life. It keeps us from becoming too aggressive and feeling too much pain, helps us learn and remember, relaxes our bodies so we can sleep, and lets us dream.

Although serotonin is involved in pretty much everything we do, think, or feel, its main role is to inhibit, to keep our warming neurotransmitters from getting out of control, to cool them off before they overheat. Serotonin gets some help from another neurotransmitter: gamma-aminobutyric acid (GABA), which is involved with regulating our central nervous system and helps us control our anxiety.

Rachel's Story: Cooling Deficiency and Obsessive-Compulsive Disorder

Jay had a patient, Rachel, who was a twenty-three-year-old Hasidic Jew with OCD. When she came into the office, she was extremely jittery. Several times during the initial consultation she got up to wash her hands, apologizing all the while. When she wasn't washing, she was eyeing the sink nervously, as though she was afraid it would disappear.

Rachel's obsessions and compulsions had started almost ten

years earlier, when she was about fourteen and became worried that she was mispronouncing words or making other mistakes when she was praying. So she started praying for longer and longer stretches of time. After a few weeks her morning prayers were nearly running together with her afternoon prayers. Her most fervent wish was that her anxiety would go away.

A few years later, as if her prayers had been answered, Rachel's compulsion to pray disappeared almost as suddenly as it had appeared. Unfortunately, it was replaced by an over-whelming fear that she wasn't completely evacuating when she relieved herself in the bathroom. So, as with the prayers, she spent longer and longer on the toilet—often as long as two hours. Then she'd leave, only to return a few minutes later. Her toilet compulsions lasted a few years and were replaced by an obses-sion with listening to the radio, afraid that she'd miss something. This one got so bad that Rachel actually quit her job so she could stay home and listen to the radio. And then the hand washing started—she washed dozens, if not hundreds of times a day, often until her hands were raw.

Because OCD is linked with cooling deficiencies, Jay prescribed a serotonin-enhancing drug, which Rachel took religiously. After a few months she felt so good that she stopped taking the drug on her own. But six months later the symptoms returned, worse than before. And this time the serotonin-enhancing drugs—Paxil, Prozac, or any others—had no effect. Jay then tried Risperdal, a dopamine blocker, which eventually relieved the symptoms.

GABA

GABA plays a particularly important role in our brains, where it mod-erates cell-to-cell communication. If it didn't, the excitatory synapses would never know when to stop firing and would eventually overheat, possibly causing a seizure. GABA-enhancing drugs are frequently used to treat epilepsy, and insufficient amounts of it have been connected to panic attacks and to conditions such as Huntington's disease, which is marked by uncontrollable, jerky movements.

When our GABA levels are balanced, we feel relaxed, comfortable in our relationships and where we are in life. Too little, though, and our world shrinks—we collect problems and the thought of any kind of change or separation becomes unbearable. Too much can disrupt our memories and cause cognitive dysfunction by keeping the cells in our brains from communicating with each other.

What we call serotonin and GABA the Ayurvedic healers called water. The analogy couldn't be more accurate. As water does to fire, serotonin and GABA do to us—they literally cool us, lubricating our brains to reduce the friction and heat of the excitatory NTs. Serotonin also plays a major role in our circulatory system; our inhibitory NTs enable us to conserve our energy and strength.

The symptoms of a person diagnosed as having "too much water" are essentially the same as those of someone with an excess of cooling NTs: boredom, lethargy, laziness, lack of motivation, low sex drive, tendency to oversleep (conserving too much energy); weight gain, obesity, greed (conserving too many things, including money and calories); being resistant to change and the unfamiliar (conserving the status quo, being unable to go with the flow); fluid retention, excessive sweating, and even dreams of water or drowning (too much liquid flowing through the system).

The symptoms of "not enough water" or a cooling deficit are fascinating—and the connections just as clear: dry mouth and constant thirst (clearly a lack of lubrication); lack of sweat and heat intolerance (lowered ability to cool); kidney stones, constipation, phlegm, congestion, and blood clots (liquids flowing too slowly).

Like the ancient Vedics, the Chinese used water or cool/wet to describe the symptoms we now associate with cooling NT deficiencies. They also associated those traits with yin (feminine, the opposite of yang, which is masculine), an element (in this case metal, which expands and contracts depending on how hot it gets), and a bodily organ—in this case two: the brain, which controls all the body's activities and functions, and the kidneys, which, like cooling NTs, clear our systems of the toxins and impurities left by the warming neurotransmitters.

Throughout the rest of this chapter we'll discuss symptoms of cooling neurotransmitter imbalances. If you haven't taken the test in chapter 2, we urge you to do so now. While you may be able to determine whether you have a deficiency or excess of serotonin or GABA by comparing the symptoms listed here with your own, we've designed the test to provide a far more accurate diagnosis of your individual imbalances.

Cooling Deficiencies and Your Mind and Body

This section will discuss how a deficiency of cooling neurotransmitters may affect your mood, cognition, behavior, and body. Keep in mind as you're reading that categorizing symptoms isn't easy. Is feeling angry all the time and lashing out at other people physically a cognitive or physical disorder? If you drink or take drugs because you're feeling depressed, is that behavior or mood? In the sections that follow, we'll take a detailed look at how cooling NT deficits affect your mind, your body, and your behavior. Although serotonin and GABA affect all three of these areas, their origins, distribution networks, and effects, and the symptoms they produce, are often subtly different. For the remainder of this chapter, though, we'll use the word *cooling* to refer to the two of them together, except when we need to discuss a specific one separately.

Your cooling neurotransmitters play a vital role in everything that goes on inside your brain. They regulate your mood and emotions, they control your memory and your ability to concentrate and learn, and they provide protection, keeping the brain safe and secure so that it can repair itself and adapt to new information. Let's take a more detailed look at the effects of low levels of any or all of the cooling NTs on a few of these areas.

All of your neurotransmitters have different—but equally important—functions in your ability to learn, focus, and remember, and in your brain's overall ability to function. Symptoms of cooling deficits include:

- memory loss
- intrusive thoughts
- inability to get negative images and memories out of your mind
- autism and schizophrenia

GABA and serotonin walk a very thin line when it comes to brain function, memory, and learning. On one hand, they (particularly GABA, which is our most important cooling neurotransmitter), are found in about 75 percent of all the synapses in the brain and facilitate somewhere between 20 and 40 percent of all communication between neurons, helping messages get where they need to go when they need to get there. On the other hand, they inhibit excess communication, which protects the neurons by keeping the heating neurotransmitter from flooding the brain with messages.

Besides being a neurotransmitter, serotonin also acts as a kind of nerve growth agent, regulating the development of brain cells. Animal studies have shown that fetuses who are exposed to serotonin-blocking drugs in utero are born with retarded brain growth. It appears that GABA, in a dynamic relationship with the warming NTs (in particular dopamine and norepinephrine), modulates thought, anxiety, and mood, while serotonin acts as a stabilizing agent, acting to return the brain to its original or *homeostatic* state.

GABA and serotonin also calm the mind, enabling you to concentrate and focus. There are major concentrations of GABA neurons, for example, in the hippocampus, a part of the brain that is involved in memory and cognitive function. When everything is working fine, cooling neurotransmitters facilitate learning by helping make short-term memories and new experiences into long-term memories. But when levels are abnormally low, your memory is affected.

Glutamate is the principal neurotransmitter involved in memory. When GABA and serotonin levels are too low to keep glutamate levels in check, new memories can't be formed. Adequate GABA and serotonin levels are necessary to keep glutamate from bombarding our brains with unpleasant thoughts. Anxiety and *post-traumatic stress disorder* (PTSD), one of the anxiety disorders, are both marked by intense recollections of disturbing images from the past. Both are also associated with low levels of GABA and serotonin.

In extreme situations, excess glutamate or a GABA deficit allows brain cells to get overstimulated, which releases even more heating neurotransmitters. This destroys otherwise healthy brain cells and can lead to anxiety, seizures, and even epilepsy. Drugs that enhance inhibition, such as most of the effective antiepileptic and antiseizure drugs, work by increasing GABA activity.

Depression and Cooling Deficiency

Normal levels of serotonin make life feel worth living. Low levels cause us to look at the world through mud-covered glasses. The lower our serotonin levels, the less control we have over our emotions and the less content we are. Patients with low levels of cooling neurotransmitters, what we call *serotonin-deficiency syndrome,* often come into our offices with some or all of the following core symptoms:

- feeling depressed or suicidal
- frequently anxious, nervous, or panicky and/or relying on tranquilizers to calm down
- worrying excessively
- persistent phobias or fears
- having a tendency to think negative thoughts
- intensely disliking change
- tending to hold grudges
- being frequently upset, irritable, annoyed, or angry
- tending to act rigidly, getting locked into a particular course of action

There's a lot of discussion among researchers and clinicians about the precise role serotonin plays in our moods and depression. Some believe that serotonin is directly responsible for causing happiness, contentment, and confidence when it's there, and anxiety, depression, and insecurity when it's not. Others believe that it only enhances those states by its absence or its presence.

The jury's still out on that one, but two things are absolutely sure:

1. Besides affecting mood, depression can lead to physical problems such as fatigue, pain that seems to have no apparent cause, poor immune system function, and increased susceptibility to allergies and disease (we'll talk more about all of these symptoms below).
2. Increasing serotonin production goes a long way to relieving these and other problems.

When we talk about depression, we usually think of a mood problem created by an emotional issue. Someone hurt our feelings, or we were disappointed by the loss of a job or a relationship, and we become depressed. There are actually millions of reasons why we get depressed, but just about everyone with depression has one thing in common—we lack the energy or warmth in our brain to maintain internal functions and a positive outlook on the world.

When most people experience something that gets them angry, frustrated, or disappointed, their brain releases tremendous amounts of dopamine, which is immediately converted into norepinephrine, the brain's adrenalin. The conversion happens so quickly that dopamine doesn't have a chance to act in its pleasure-enhancing capacity. As norepinephrine floods the brain, it increases alertness, vigilance, and reactivity. All this action heats the brain, causing inflammation, which results in the release of another chemical that's involved in alertness: histamine. The norepinephrine-histamine combination puts the brain on high alert.

In an effort to protect itself, the brain shuts down production of warming neurotransmitters. The first thing to go is our positive outlook; the second is motor activity and mental acuity, which makes us feel, look, and act "depressed." Interestingly, depressed patients frequently have heightened levels of acetylcholine, another warming neurotransmitter that is intimately involved in motor activity. This may explain the agitated state and disturbed sleep patterns these patients so often report. If the shutdown lasts a day or so, you get the blues. If it goes on for weeks or months, you get chronic or major depression.

Now here's the twist: warmth and motivation can't exist without cooling and safety. And if serotonin levels are too low, the brain won't turn dopamine production back on. Think of a deer caught in the headlights of your car. It's scared and its brain has released a huge jolt of dopamine that makes the deer's heart race and its breathing shallow and quick. But it still can't move. The overload of dopamine paralyzed the deer. A few seconds later, when the deer's brain releases a little serotonin, the deer can bolt out of the road and back into the forest. In people the mechanism is basically the same. Increase the baseline levels of cooling neurotransmitters and you restore levels of warming activity. The SSRIs (which we'll talk more about later) increase cooling and enable the brain to warm itself. Remember, though, that health, function, comfort, and well-being are not simply the result of high levels of warming or cooling neurotransmitters. Instead, they are the result of a delicate balance between the two.

If you don't examine and process the original thoughts, events, or emotions that caused the hyperexcitation, the cycle will repeat itself and you'll get even more depressed. The treatment is usually to increase the dosage of medication, but that ultimately fails. Lasting success can only be achieved by restoring balance and resolving the original source of excitation.

Depression is an equal-opportunity condition. Although conventional psychological wisdom has it that more women than men suffer from depression, we believe that men's refusal to admit that they may have a problem may be skewing the statistics.

Stress and Anxiety and Cooling Deficiency

Stress is extremely important in our lives. It makes us pay attention, keeps us on our toes, enables us to think clearly and to stay focused. During times of stress, the hypothalamus releases a hormone called *corticotropin-releasing factor* (CRF), which coordinates the body's response to stress and helps it prepare for the danger it perceives. It heats up our circuits, raising our blood pressure, increasing our heart rate, and telling our metabolism to burn more glucose for fuel. It also stimulates the heating neurons in our brain, which is what causes increased arousal and vigilance. CRF has a direct effect on the immune system, increasing the release of molecules called *inflammatory cytokines,* which tell the immune system to get ready to fight (see "Your Immune System" below). In animal studies, CRF has been shown to increase motor activity, negative emotionality (growling and hissing), and conflict behavior (picking fights, etc.).

A little stress and a little CRF go a long way. Theoretically, our cooling neurotransmitters, GABA and serotonin, help cool off our hypothalamic panic button, naturally slowing down the body's emergency response reaction by inhibiting the release of CRF. When a stressful situation lasts for more than a few days or is too intense, we can't produce enough GABA and serotonin to put out the fire. The result can be muscle tension, exaggerated startle responses, irritability, high blood pressure, stomach problems, and more. If we stay in a stressful state for a few *months,* the symptoms get worse and may include chest pains, panic attacks, and severe depression.

Like stress, anxiety is a perfectly normal, self-protective reaction to threatening situations. And like stress, a little anxiety goes a long way. Too much, and you become unnecessarily fearful, apprehensive, nervous, panicky, restless, and likely to perceive ordinary situations as dangerous or threatening. It's often described as a generalized response to an unknown threat or internal conflict. Physical symptoms include trembling, fainting, headaches, and sweating.

Ricky Williams's Story: Cooling Deficiency and Social Anxiety

Ricky Williams was always in the spotlight. As a running back at the University of Texas, he won the Heisman Trophy. In 1999 he became one of the hottest commodities in the pro football draft. Mike Ditka, who was the head coach of the New Orleans Saints, traded the team's entire draft to get Williams. The media barrage that followed Williams completely overwhelmed him.

He never seemed able to play up to expectations. He ran away from autograph-seeking fans and kept his helmet strapped to his head during interviews. "It got to the point where I didn't want to leave my house," he was quoted as saying. "I was afraid of situations where I actually had to talk to someone." He stopped shopping, couldn't date, hated to travel, and even backed out of public appearances. People thought he was nuts, and the Saints traded him to the Miami Dolphins.

Ricky finally met with a therapist who diagnosed him with social anxiety disorder and prescribed Paxil, an SSRI. In what seems like a miraculous turnaround, Williams became one of the stars of the Miami offense and now eagerly participates in public appearances. "I've become a better person, I've become a better father, I've become a better teammate," he said in an interview with the Associated Press. "It's just the greatest feeling in the whole wide world."

Panic Disorder

Panic disorder takes everything up another notch. It typically begins out of the blue, with feelings of impending doom and fear. Symptoms often include chest pains, fear of going crazy, numbness, and the feeling of being smothered.

When CRF is released, so is the warming neurotransmitter glutamate, too much of which can cause brain damage even when there hasn't been any physical injury. Several studies have shown that people or animals who had long-term exposure to significant stressors, such as parental deprivation, child abuse, or being reared in isolation, had excessive levels of glutamate. We know that patients suffering from depression, anxiety, and panic disorders have measurably increased levels of CRF. Researchers are currently developing antianxiety and antidepression drugs that are CRF antagonists, meaning that they block CRF release.

Post-Traumatic Stress Disorder and Cooling Deficiency

Frank was a forty-seven-year-old police officer. He was obese, had a flushed complexion and a sour look on his face, was short of breath, and winced in pain with almost every step he took. Just a few days before his first visit with Jay he'd gotten into a fight with a coworker outside the precinct. He experienced sudden chest pains, almost collapsed, and was taken to the hospital, where he had a cardiac workup that came back normal. That's when he was referred to Jay's office.

At first, all Frank wanted to talk about were his physical symptoms—especially the pain. Low back pain, chest pain, pain while walking, pain while sitting. And then, of course, there was the racing heart, the diarrhea, the night sweats, and the overwhelming fatigue. Amazingly, most of these symptoms had been going on for eight years. But over the previous year things had gotten worse. He'd been eating compulsively and had put on forty pounds. He'd seen a number of specialists, including a gastroenterologist who thought he had irritable bowel syndrome, but the medication he prescribed didn't alleviate those symptoms.

At one point during the exam, Jay asked Frank what the fight was about. Reluctantly he explained that eight years before, he'd stopped at a supermarket one evening after work. He was maybe twenty feet from the checkout line when a man pulled a gun on the clerk. Even though he was off duty, Frank was carrying a gun. But he froze. He tried to move and tried to react but he couldn't. Before fleeing, the gunman shot three other customers, one of whom landed, dead, just a few feet away from Frank.

For a few days he was angry at himself. As a cop he'd been trained to react under pressure, but when the chips were down he'd choked. Then the nightmares started. He'd wake up screaming, pulse racing, the sheets drenched. Things weren't much better when he was awake, as he replayed the holdup in his mind over and over and over, hundreds of times a day. He started missing a lot of work, and even when he was there he couldn't concentrate and felt as though he were outside himself watching instead of actually being there. His performance at work led to friction with his partners and to an occasional fight outside the precinct.

Jay started Frank on a regimen of folic acid, omega-3 fatty acids, and magnesium. That took the edge off some of the symptoms, but there was still a long way to go. The next step was a prescription for Zoloft, a serotonin-enhancing drug that is often used as an antidepressant and that is FDA-approved for treating post-traumatic stress disorder (PTSD). After about three weeks, Frank's irritable bowel problems had all but disappeared and he started to smile again—for the first time in years. Over the course of the next few months, his other symptoms also decreased to manageable levels.

◆ ◆ ◆

PTSD typically follows a particularly stressful event, one that often involves a real or perceived threat to life. The victim reexperiences the event over and over again, in different ways, including intrusive thoughts, flashbacks, and vivid dreams. Untreated, patients with PTSD can develop persistently high levels of sympathetic nervous system activity, including high blood pressure, increased pulse, etc. They also have been shown to have brain damage, a literal shrinking of certain areas of the brain, particularly the hippocampus, which governs memory and the perception of pain.

Ordinarily, the brain is in a constant state of change because new experiences and memories physically change its structure by creating new pathways between neurons. But in cases of extreme stress such as PTSD, glutamate suppresses the process by which neurons regenerate, and the effect is that the brain is essentially flash frozen. The negative images and memories are permanently burned into the brain, which is why they keep coming back. In addition, the ability to form new memories (or to forget old ones) is inhibited.

About 9 percent of those exposed to trauma will develop PTSD. Several studies, however, have shown that the risk for women is about twice as high as for men (13 percent vs. 6 percent). Not surprisingly, in the months following the terrorist attacks on the World Trade Center, New Yorkers were experiencing PTSD at twice the national rate.

Obsessive-Compulsive Disorder and Cooling Deficiency

Obsessive-compulsive disorder (OCD) is really a two-part disease consisting of obsessions (unwanted urges or ideas, such as a fear of becoming contaminated, worries of hurting someone or of being hurt, or a need to be perfect or to make everything symmetrical) and compulsions (endlessly repetitive behavior that is supposed to reduce the anxiety that the obsession causes, such as washing the hands, repeatedly checking to see whether doors are locked, counting, arranging, cleaning, or hoarding). It has been shown that repeating familiar actions such as chewing or rocking increases cooling NTs.

OCD is considered a *spectrum disorder,* meaning that it might include other conditions such as eating disorders, Tourette's syndrome, and trichotillomania (compulsive hair pulling). People suffering from this imbalance are driven to think things they don't want to think and do things they don't want to do because of a deficiency of the cooling NTs that would otherwise restrain them. This might include anything from simply being superstitious to far more complex and incapacitating compulsions such as washing one's body raw or refusing to go to sleep because of the need to do things like checking to see whether the stove burners are off or the front door is locked, over and over again.

Although it's clear that one of the biological bases of OCD is a deficit of serotonin, only 60 percent of patients respond positively to serotonin-enhancing medication. This indicates that other neurotransmitters, along with stress-related adrenal chemicals called *glucocorticoids* (more on them below), may contribute to the problem. Dopamine excess, for example, is known to cause tics and other OCD-like behaviors.

Body Function and Cooling Deficiency

As already noted, seizures such as those associated with epilepsy are caused by a deficiency of GABA, a cooling neurotransmitter that modulates the flow of information and keeps communication between neurons from becoming excessive. Ballet dancers who seem so calm and effortless while moving in and out of graceful contortions, yoga aficionados relaxing in near impossible poses, and even your favorite NFL quarterback going deep for the receiver in the end zone are relying heavily on GABA to keep them calm and their movements coordinated under pressure.

GABA is vital in two distinct areas of movement: the jaw and the eyes. Impairing the neurons that release and respond to GABA makes it nearly impossible for a patient to control his or her jaw while chewing and swallowing. In addition, sleep researchers have found that GABA, the overseer of sleep, coordinates the movements of the eyes during the most vivid form of dreaming, REM sleep. GABA also coordinates and maintains respiration during sleep. The marked differences between the rhythm and periodicity of wakefulness and sleep are the result of the relative predominance of GABA. This has added significance when evaluating sleep disorders such as insomnia, early-morning or middle-of-the-night awakening, and the impact they have on daytime fatigue and attentiveness.

PMS and Cooling Deficiency

Typically, women have lowered serotonin levels before and during menstruation, which in part explains why many women feel anxious, depressed, and angry, or suffer from migraines—all symptoms of low GABA and/or serotonin. It also may explain why women often experience particularly strong cravings for chocolate and carbohydrates, both of which increase cooling NTs. Researchers have found that treating women suffering from PMS with the cooling neurotransmitter–enhancing drug d-fenfluramine before menstruation and just after its onset significantly reduces premenstrual depression and decreases carbohydrate cravings and intake by 40 percent. In clinical practice, another group of serotonin-enhancing drugs, the SSRIs, are often used to treat PMS.

PMDD

Premenstrual dysphoric disorder (PMDD) is a particularly serious form of PMS that affects about 5 percent of women in the second half of their cycle. Symptoms include clinical depression, anxiety, and irritability, but they go way beyond those of ordinary PMS. A recent study published in the *Archives of General Psychiatry* found a strong connection between GABA deficits and PMDD. One of GABA's many functions is to reduce feelings of pain and anxiety by slowing down communication between mood-related nerve cells. Women with PMDD have been shown to have lower GABA and serotonin levels than women who don't.

Your Heart and Cooling Deficiency

There's a growing field of medicine called *neurocardiology,* which recognizes that the heart and the brain are related more intimately than any other two organs in the body. When catastrophic events such as earthquakes, hurricanes, or terrorist attacks hit, among the casualties are always people who weren't actually injured by the event but suffered fatal heart attacks.

Researchers have identified some specific personality traits that predispose one to heart disease, and no, it's not the Type A personality, which was recently disproved as a heart attack risk. *Type D* (for distressed) people are characterized by negative emotions, including hostility, increased tendency to worry, frequently feeling unhappy or irritated, and being easily provoked to anger. In our practice we call this particular constellation of symptoms a *serotonin deficiency state*.

Having negative emotions is one thing. But how you deal with those feelings can also have a significant impact on the development of heart disease.

Hostility increases the risk of heart disease sevenfold. People who are hostile release increased amounts of norepinephrine into the bloodstream. (Some researchers have dubbed these people "hot reactors"—people whose blood pressure seems normal at rest but shoots up to dangerously high levels during stress.) They have excessive heart rate reactivity and may also have an exaggerated heart response to relatively innocuous events.

A number of other personality traits influence heart disease and heart attack risk as well. Patients suffering from depression have four times the risk of developing heart disease than the general population (20 percent vs. 5 percent). Those whose depression is untreated have significantly higher risk of dying of a cardiovascular condition than those who aren't depressed or whose depression is being treated. Major depression is considered by doctors to be a better indicator than diabetes or hypertension of a patient's risk of dying of a heart attack.

Researchers have discovered that in people who already have low serotonin, stress and anxiety release adrenaline, which kicks the immune system into action, making it respond as if there's an actual injury that needs repair. White blood cells stream into the arteries, where they interact with cholesterol and create a mucky substance (plaque) that hardens and builds up inside the arteries, ultimately leading to heart disease or heart attack. People with normal serotonin levels don't have that reaction when stressed. Lowering stress levels and cholesterol can help reduce the risk of this dangerous cascade of events.

People with panic disorder usually have overly high levels of warming neurotransmitters, especially norepinephrine. Symptoms include anxiety, tremors, increased heart rate, and excessive sweating. The result is an increased tendency to form blood clots and a greater chance of developing *cardiac arrhythmia* (irregular heartbeat). In addition, people with untreated anxiety are three times more likely to have heart disease than the general population.

A variety of studies have shown that stress can cause sudden cardiac death. Sudden cardiac death is caused by a sudden spike in some warming, fight-or-flight chemicals, such as adrenaline, without the adequate counterbalancing effect of the cooling neurotransmitters.

Actually, the spikes of warming neurotransmitters and other chemicals by themselves do *not* cause heart attacks. The more serious problem is a deficiency of cooling neurotransmitters that leaves the warming neurotransmitters, particularly norepinephrine, unopposed. This increases heart rate, blood pressure, spasm of coronary arteries, likelihood that platelets will clot, and risk of cardiac arrhythmias.

A number of studies have shown that patients with no known heart condition who were taking serotonin-boosting drugs to control depression, anxiety, panic disorders, and other noncardiac conditions were far less likely to have heart attacks than those who weren't taking them.

Allergies and Asthma and Cooling Deficiency

Allergies, asthma, osteoarthritis, recurrent or chronic congestion, heartburn, sore throats, sinus or upper respiratory infections, aches, pains, and stiffness make up the majority of complaints family doctors deal with. Most doctors interpret symptoms like these as inflammatory and order a few tests. If the tests come back positive for bacterial infection, they prescribe antibiotics, which usually work well.

But too often, the tests come back negative and doctors prescribe antibiotics anyway, assuming that an undetectable bacteria is responsible. The problem with that approach is that in a lot of cases, those conditions really are not allergies, asthma, or arthritis but the result of an excess of warming neurotransmitters that causes an inflammatory immune system reaction severe enough and long-lasting enough to produce symptoms. In cases like this, antibiotics don't work or make the condition worse.

The problem is that many antibiotics mimic the effect of the cooling neurotransmitters. Taking them for a few days ends up creating a state of cooling excess, or warming deficiency, which slows the immune system and leaves the body susceptible to infection and illness. It leaves you feeling exhausted and achy.

Pain and Cooling Deficiency

Pain is a critical part of our existence; it's the brain's way of telling us to stop doing something that could be dangerous or harmful. But too much pain can cause tissue damage and inflammation—and it makes life miserable.

Sensations of pain are determined by two types of cells in the spinal cord that receive sensory information from all over the body and transmit it to the brain: *on* and *off* cells. On cells activate in response to something painful, such as touching your hand to a hot stove. Glutamate coordinates and transmits on-cell signals within the brain. Off cells, which are coordinated by serotonin and GABA, slow down transmission of pain by reducing signals from the spinal cord to the brain. Off cells are activated by painkillers, particularly opiates such as Percocet (oxycodone), morphine, and codeine.

One of GABA's main functions is to keep messages from traveling between cells too quickly. This helps reduce anxiety and nervousness and cravings for food or drugs. It also reduces the perception of pain by keeping too many messages from reaching the brain, letting them through only when there's really something to worry about. When there isn't enough GABA around to do the job, though, sensitivity to pain goes way up. The body responds by sending what little GABA it has left to deal with the situation, but that just depletes GABA further and makes the pain worse.

Studies measuring relative concentrations of glutamate and GABA in the brain have shown that people suffering from chronic pain conditions including fibromyalgia have significantly higher glutamate and lower GABA levels than pain-free controls.

When glutamate receptors are stimulated, they release calcium into the surrounding brain cells. This releases a pro-inflammatory fatty acid called *arachidonic acid,* which facilitates learning and brain–body communication. But too much arachidonic acid has some extremely dangerous consequences, including destructive immune system activation, increased pain transmission, increased blood clotting, decreased blood flow, and brain inflammation. Together, these symptoms are called an *arachidonic acid cascade.*

Recent research by the National Institutes of Mental Health speculated that one of the ways many of the anticonvulsive medications work is by inhibiting arachidonic acid, which cools the brain and reduces heat and inflammation. Recent studies have demonstrated that drugs that block inflammation, such as Celebrex, may be helpful in patients with schizophrenia (another excess-heat state) when used in conjunction with typical antipsychotic medications. Dr. Andrew Stoll at Harvard has demonstrated that high doses of omega-3 fatty acids (which reduce arachidonic acid by reducing the relative levels of omega-6 fats) are helpful for bipolar patients.

Migraines and
Cooling Deficiency

Recent studies have shown that migraine headaches are associated with a state of *cortical hyperexcitability* (meaning that brain cells are overactive), which is caused by a lack of *intracortical inhibition* (meaning that the mechanisms for reducing excess communication within the brain aren't functioning). In simpler terms, there's either too much glutamate or not enough GABA to calm things down. During the actual migraine attack, magnesium levels drop, which further excites the cells. Taking daily magnesium supplements has been demonstrated to reduce headache frequency. Recent evidence indicates that 5-HTP, an over-the-counter serotonin booster, can have dramatic effects on both the duration and the intensity of severe headaches and migraines.

Many of the common prescription drugs used to treat chronic migraines, including Depakote and Topamax, are really antiseizure medications that work by increasing GABA or decreasing glutamate. For acute migraines, drugs in the *triptan* family, such as Imitrex and Maxalt, relieve the pain by regulating serotonin receptors on the cranial arteries, which in turn reduces the inflammation in the blood vessels.

Fibromyalgia and
Cooling Deficiency

Fibromyalgia (FM) is a chronic pain condition, which, like all other chronic pain conditions, is due either to an excess of glutamate (which amplifies the intensity and speed of pain messages) or a decrease in serotonin or GABA function, both of which slow down pain message transmission. Besides excruciating and debilitating muscle pain, FM patients often experience depression and sleep disturbances related to cooling deficits. In addition, researchers are investigating links between FM and migraines and irritable bowel syndrome. The most successful treatments for FM are serotonin- and GABA-enhancing drugs.

For the past few decades, a small number of researchers have been exploring a possible connection between fibromyalgia and sleep disturbances. One of the pioneers of this research, the Canadian psychiatrist Harvey Moldofsky, has suggested that fibromyalgia results from a deficiency of circulating tryptophan (which the brain uses to make serotonin). That deficiency interferes with the patient's slow-wave sleep. It's during this period of sleep that the brain releases hormones that stimulate the repair and regeneration of the body's tissues. Without enough slow-wave sleep, tissue never gets a chance to heal properly, and the constant irritation results in the pain that plagues fibromyalgia sufferers.

Pain and Depression and Cooling Deficiency

There's no question that pain—especially chronic pain—and depression are intertwined and that each condition aggravates the other. One recent study of 19,000 subjects in several European countries found that depressed people were four times more likely to have chronic pain than nondepressed patients. In the United States, over 75 percent of patients who see their primary care physician for depression also complain of headaches; stomach, neck, or back pain; musculoskeletal pain, chest pain, and hard-to-locate pain or generalized pain, according to Maurizio Fava, director of the Depression Clinic at Massachusetts General Hospital in Boston.

The worse a person's pain and the longer it lasts, the greater the risk for depression. Chronic pain has also been linked with immune system suppression, fatigue, and reduced physical performance.

Depression and increased pain sensitivity are both caused by the same inadequate levels of cooling neurotransmitters in the brain. Sometimes that deficiency gets expressed as pain, other times as depression, and quite often as both. Confirming that connection is the fact that Prozac and other serotonin-boosting medications have been shown to reduce pain as well as depressive symptoms. On the nonprescription front, 5-HTP is quite effective in improving both conditions.

Your Skin and Cooling Deficiency

Most people don't think of their skin as a sensory organ, but it is—in fact, it's the biggest organ in your body. And as an organ, it is connected to and influenced by your thoughts, feelings, and emotions. Just think of the goose bumps you get at a scary movie or the way you blush when you get embarrassed.

These and many more serious skin conditions are caused by cooling NT deficits or warming excesses, such as those brought on by allergic reaction or a negative reaction to certain drugs. The common manifestations of some of them make the connection obvious. Psoriasis, for example, is marked by inflamed, hot, red, dry, and itchy skin, usually on the scalp, lower back, knees, and elbows. Other skin conditions, such as rashes, acne, and eczema are also red, inflamed, and irritated— clearly an excess of heat.

Exactly when a dermatologic problem first appears and how long it lasts is greatly influenced by stress, anxiety, or other psychological condition. Herpes is often triggered by stress, and researchers have found strong connections between psoriasis and social phobia, and between acne and obsessive-compulsive disorder. (Keep in mind that stress and other conditions only make skin conditions worse; they don't cause them.)

Dermatologists typically treat skin conditions with topical drugs or antibiotics without regard to the possibly underlying causes. Those familiar with the relatively new field of psychodermatology, however, recognize that managing patients' dermatological condition often requires dealing with their emotional and psychological issues. In many cases, serious skin conditions can be cleared up with serotonin-boosting antidepressants and/or anti-anxiety medication.

Irritable Bowel Syndrome and Cooling Deficiency

Irritable bowel syndrome, gas, cramps, and other stomach problems— while the expression, "You are what you eat" may not be precisely true, "You feel what you eat" certainly is. In truth, there's a very strong connection between the stomach and the brain. Stimulating the intestines triggers the release of histamines (inflammatory chemicals) in the brain—especially the limbic system, which is the seat of memory and emotion. This may explain why many clinicians claim that patients with chronic gastrointestinal problems are more depressed and have worse overall mental health than patients with any other chronic disease.

Alcohol and Cooling Deficiency

If you've ever felt the glow of a martini or a margarita, you understand what it feels like to increase your cooling neurotransmitters. As discussed above, a drink every now and then may be good for you. But when it goes from a nice way to kick back and relax to a "gotta have it" substance, you're in trouble.

Between alcohol, cigarettes, and illicit drugs, there are over 75 million addicts in the United States—enough to qualify as a real epidemic. And if we include obesity from addictive sugar and carbohydrate intake, the problem is much bigger. Researchers have recently discovered that there may be a genetic predisposition to addiction. Not surprisingly, that predisposition is mirrored in a shift in the balance between warming and cooling neurotransmitters. Addictions are a person's attempt to self-medicate—to restore neurotransmitter balance—but the type of addiction depends to a great extent on the direction of the imbalance.

A serotonin-deficient person might try to increase his or her cooling NT levels by giving in to chocolate cravings or going on carbohydrate eating binges, both of which *briefly* increase serotonin. A GABA-deficient person would be more likely to take tranquilizers (such as Valium, Xanax, or Ativan) or to be an alcoholic, since those substances themselves increase GABA levels in the brain. As a cooling neurotransmitter, GABA slows down activity, which explains the typical symptoms of drunkenness—slurred speech, slowed reaction time, impaired coordination, and so on. Long-term alcohol consumption gradually makes GABA receptors less sensitive, meaning that you need to drink more to get the same effect.

Excessive drinking, by keeping GABA levels high and glutamate levels low, keeps alcoholics' brains in a constant state of sedation. But when an alcoholic suddenly stops drinking, the absence of GABA leads to a sudden excess of glutamate, which overstimulates the brain. The result is often unpleasant, and includes nausea, restlessness, insomnia, anxiety, sometimes even the DTs *(delirium tremens),* seizures, hallucinations, or psychotic behavior—all symptoms of warming excess/cooling deficit.

Serotonin also plays an important role in alcoholism. Alcohol increases the cooling-deficient person's serotonin levels up to normal by triggering the release of serotonin from brain cells. But there isn't much serotonin in the brain cells to begin with, so they're quickly depleted. This makes the alcoholic drink even more in a futile attempt to boost serotonin in his brain. Researchers have come up with two scenarios for how this can play out.

1. Someone whose serotonin levels are always low will drink every day in order to feel better.

2. For some people, alcohol doesn't release enough serotonin to restore balance. Without enough serotonin to tell them they've had enough, binge drinkers sometimes don't put down their beers until they pass out.

Other Addictive Behaviors and Cooling Deficiency

Marijuana.   Like caffeine, marijuana triggers a serotonin release in the brain. This makes the smoker feel better. But after a short while, serotonin levels get depleted and that feeling of safety fades, often to be replaced by paranoia and hunger. Since marijuana doesn't have any noticeable impact on dopamine or the brain's pleasure centers, it technically isn't an addictive drug. However, by making serotonin deficiencies worse, it can make the dope smoker more susceptible to trying—and becoming addicted to—other drugs.

Ecstasy.   Ecstasy doesn't have much of an effect on dopamine, but it releases all of the brain's serotonin at the same time, filling the user with overwhelming feelings of warmth, safety, and love for everyone and everything. Many Ecstasy users report that the drug acts like an aphrodisiac, increasing their desire to have sex. However, like many prescription serotonin-enhancing drugs, Ecstasy often has sexual side effects, including an inability to reach orgasm. The serotonin drain is so complete that people can be depressed for days after they take the drug. Repeated use can cause permanent damage to the serotonin receptors.

Oniomania.   This is the medical term for "shop till you drop" or shopaholism. Unfortunately, shopaholism is usually relegated to joke punch lines, but the fact is that it can be a serious condition. Oniomania is an obsessive, addictive disorder. Compulsive shoppers (who have been shown to be serotonin deficient) lack the self-control to stop themselves from spending money. Like other addicts, they give in to their irresistible urges. This condition can be devastating, leading to depression and anxiety, divorce, bankruptcy, and embezzlement. Estimates are that 8–10 percent of Americans are shopaholics—80–90 percent of them women (as are 80 percent of kleptomaniacs, who also can't control their urges). Female oniomaniacs tend to spend their money on makeup and jewelry, while men buy high-tech gadgets.

Food Cravings and Obesity and Cooling Deficiency

Because eating is so critical to our survival, there may be more than one cause for the mechanisms that trigger hunger and food cravings. Generally speaking, obesity is a warming-deficiency condition; however, a fascinating paper recently published in the journal *Nutrition* suggested that it may be exactly the opposite—an inflammatory disease caused by a cooling deficit. The study's authors found that overweight children and adults had elevated inflammatory *cytokines*, which are associated with dopamine-excess/serotonin-deficient immune cell activity. They also hypothesized that the pandemic prevalence of obesity today might be the result of insufficient breast-feeding and the absence of anti-inflammatory fatty acids in the diet of infants.

Obesity specialists often say that their patients can't "beat the cortisol," meaning that they have great difficulty losing body fat, especially from around the waist, while under stress. This resistance to weight and body fat loss is the direct and indirect result of elevated cortisol and inflammation. Cholesterol-lowering statin drugs as well as foods and supplements containing fatty acids help lower this resistance, but the only way to truly reach the problem at its roots is to balance the cooling and warming NTs.

Eating Disorders and Cooling Deficiency

Lori was a sixteen-year-old girl who was referred to Jay by her pediatrician. She was about 10 percent underweight, had headaches and very irregular menstrual periods, and hadn't grown at all since she was fourteen. She described herself as shy, something of a perfectionist, and very close to her parents.

An endocrine (hormone) workup came back normal, and Jay was concerned that a tumor in the pituitary gland might be the cause of her symptoms. But when an MRI of her brain didn't show anything abnormal, he began to suspect that Lori was anorexic.

When she was fourteen, her parents' marriage started to unravel. They fought constantly, often in front of Lori. Mealtimes began to center around her refusal to eat—Lori hoped that not eating would get her parents to stop fighting. But despite her insight into her behavior, her parents eventually divorced and Lori continued to lose weight.

Jay prescribed a combination of serotonin-enhancing antidepressants and regular talk therapy. Lori's weight has stabilized and her headaches have disappeared, but she still has a long way to go.

The most common eating disorders are bulimia (marked by binge eating and purging) and anorexia (self-starvation), together affecting about 2 percent of adolescent girls and young women. Although about 80 percent of those with eating disorders are female, an increasing number of adolescent boys and young men are beginning to show symptoms.

There are two schools of thought on eating disorders. One holds that they're a psychological obsession with food. The more interesting theory is that they're an obsession with control and a product of a seriously distorted body image. Bulimic and anorexic patients usually come from highly controlled environments. The controlling influences (usually parents) threaten the person so much that she develops a cooling deficiency. That deficiency becomes so severe that it results in a warming excess that in some cases mimics the symptoms of psychosis, distorting the patient's perception and sense of reality.

In a number of fascinating studies, women with severe anorexia were asked to circle one of three drawings that they felt best illustrated their own figure. They overwhelmingly picked the moderate to obese figure. Another study asked anorexic women to draw the outline of a door that would be big enough for them to pass through. Each time, they drew an opening that was at least twice as large as they actually needed.

Anorexic patients crave control and choose starvation as their way to achieve it. Bulimic patients crave control and reward—she or he eats for reward and vomits or purges (or both) for control.

Preliminary research has shown that serotonin-enhancing drugs such as SSRIs are effective in treating a number of eating disorders.

Sleep and Cooling Deficiency

Whether you realize it or not, sleep is a complex behavior. All animals including humans need sleep to survive. There are actually two kinds of sleep. REM sleep is associated with dreaming and is essential for learning—especially for infants and children—and for resting the brain. Non-REM or NREM sleep is thought to be physiologically restorative. Serotonin and GABA are the neurotransmitters that help regulate sleep, and they do it in a way that is consistent with everything else they do: during sleep the brain's functions slow and its temperature drops. The more awake you are, the more dopamine, norepinephrine, and histamine there are in your brain; the more drowsy, the higher your GABA and serotonin levels. The specific area of the brain that controls normal sleep is called the *anterior hypothalamus,* where GABA is the reigning neurotransmitter. GABA sends signals from the anterior hypothalamus to the brain stem, which is the brain's primary wakefulness center, telling it to chill. Serotonin may promote sleep by stimulating increased GABA release. Interestingly, epileptics who are sleep deprived report an increase in seizure frequency. This makes sense because GABA decreases with wakefulness and glutamate—which can fry brain cells and cause seizures—increases.

REM sleep is a condition brought about when GABA carefully mutes all of the pathways leading to the cerebral cortex, the area of the brain where ideas and images are formed, except the dopamine pathways. By leaving these pathways lit, GABA allows the cortex to vividly see and experience all the visions of the mind's eye. Amid much debate, sleep researchers now believe that REM dreaming is actually the projection of learned material onto the cortex for sorting and organization to allow for more efficient memory storage and retrieval. It could be that's why we often remember things more clearly after a good night's sleep.

In years past scientists debated whether sleep was an active or passive state and whether it is induced or simply happens when excitatory activity in the brain is exhausted. Scientists in the nineteenth century put an end to the discussion by proving that sleep was induced and therefore an active condition of the brain. They isolated a chemical they called *hypnotoxin* from the spinal fluid of sleep-deprived dogs and injected it into a rested dog, which immediately fell asleep.

Hypnotoxin, which is now called *substance S* (for sleep), is most likely a mixture of GABA and the intermediary forms from which it is derived and into which it breaks down. The two chemicals responsible for keeping us awake and vigilant are dopamine and norepinephrine. They get a little help in resisting the sleepy effects of serotonin and GABA from an inflammatory immune chemical histamine. (The *antihistamine dyphenhydramine* is the main ingredient found in Benadryl and other popular "PM" over-the-counter cold and cough medicines and helps induce sleep.) Prescription hypnotics or sleep-inducing drugs mainly fall into the class of agents called *benzodiazepines,* of which the first was Valium. All of these drugs work by increasing GABA.

A cooling deficit can be caused either by a true shortage of a particular cooling neurotransmitter or by a relative excess of a warming NT. How do your neurotransmitters affect your sleep?

- If you need less sleep than you used to or if you have especially vivid dreams and nightmares, you probably have an excess of dopamine.
- If you have dreams of being abandoned or left alone, or if you have problems staying asleep (as opposed to falling asleep), you probably have a GABA deficiency.
- If you have insomnia or have trouble falling asleep, you probably have a serotonin deficiency.
- If you have dreams of being paralyzed or unable to run away, you have a glutamate excess.

During deep sleep—where you get most of your rest—norepinephrine levels in the brain drop, while serotonin levels rise. If you're low on serotonin, though, you may not get as much rest as you need. Sleep-deprived people can suffer from a number of cooling deficit/warming excess conditions, including:

- anxiety
- irritability
- psychosis
- hallucinations
- problems with concentration and memory
- depression
- fatigue
- sleep apnea (inability to reach deep states of sleep, resulting in hundreds of mini awakenings throughout the night)
- restless leg syndrome
- indigestion

According to the National Sleep Foundation, not getting enough sleep may also worsen conditions such as diabetes, heart disease, and arthritis in adults aged fifty-five to eighty-four. But the connection between sleep and illness is somewhat circular: while lack of sleep can exacerbate medical conditions, chronic illness can also contribute to sleep problems.

Whether your sleep issues are caused by a warming excess or a cooling deficit, the cure is to raise your cooling levels high enough to get the two back in balance.

Sex and Cooling Deficiency

Dopamine activates an area of the brain called the *septo-hippocampus*, which is integral to arousal. The hormones involved in courtship and sex depend on adequate dopamine signaling. Under normal circumstances, serotonin keeps dopamine production under control by increasing prolactin (a hormone that tends to inhibit sexual desires). The result is a normal libido. This libido can change, though, depending on the relative balance between serotonin and dopamine.

Most of us wouldn't complain if there were a slight tilt toward dopamine, which would increase interest in sex, arousal, and probably frequency of sexual activity. But if the imbalance became too great and serotonin levels fell too far, the same warming excess that contributes to heart problems, obesity, depression, and impulse control could lead to sex-related problems, particularly sexual addictions, promiscuity, tendencies to engage in risky sexual behavior, and even sexual assault.

Problems arise when patients seek treatment for other serotonin-deficiency conditions, particularly depression. Although serotonin is generally quite effective in reducing symptoms of depression, there's often a cost. About 60 percent of patients taking serotonin-enhancing drugs (SSRIs) experience some degree of sexual dysfunction, most commonly decreased arousal and an inability (or extreme difficulty) to reach orgasm.

SSRIs work by increasing the amount of serotonin in the brain, but some of these drugs wreak sexual havoc by inhibiting an enzyme called *nitric oxide*. Nitric oxide (NO) is a chemical messenger that's an ally of the warming, inflammatory neurotransmitters dopamine, norepinephrine, and acetylcholine. It's involved in a number of biological functions, including increasing blood flow to a number of critical organs. (Viagra, by the way, works by increasing NO activity, sending blood to the penis in much the same way you might inflate a balloon.) The lower the level of NO, the greater the sexual problems. This is why many psychiatrists are now augmenting prescriptions for SSRIs—which can diminish the NO effect—with small amounts of dopamine-enhancing drugs such as Wellbutrin or Viagra.

Multiple Sclerosis and Cooling Deficiency

As serotonin is metabolized by the body or brain, its major waste product is 5-HIAA. Multiple sclerosis (MS) patients have reduced levels of 5-HIAA in their urine and cerebral spinal fluid. Preliminary data suggest that MS symptoms can be eased by using drugs that either slow down the rate of serotonin metabolism (SSRIs) or increase serotonin production. In addition, reducing stress—a known trigger for MS patients—has been shown to slow down the progression of the disease.

Laurie's Story: Cooling Deficiency and MS

Laurie, forty-four, described herself as energetic and a real go-getter, but also dependent and emotionally sensitive. When she was in her early thirties she started experiencing a strange numbness in her hands. She saw a neurologist who told her not to worry about it. It wasn't until nearly a decade later that she was diagnosed with multiple sclerosis.

MS is a cooling-deficiency condition that is aggravated by stress. And Laurie had plenty of it. She was married to a man who made her feel unattractive, and their sex life was unsatisfying and infrequent.

She had just filed for a divorce, which raised her stress levels and eroded her cooling neurotransmitters even more, when she suddenly developed urinary incontinence—leaking fluid whenever she felt stressed, which was most of the time. And as if that weren't bad enough, she also became hypersensitive to heat. The slightest amount of exercise made her intensely hot, and she could wear only cotton. Any other fabrics made her skin feel like it was burning. It was as if the fluid leak was causing her system to overheat.

This went on for several months, until she began an intense sexual relationship with a younger man who made her feel beautiful and confident. The only time she was ever free from her heat sensitivity and incontinence was when she was involved in a deep, emotional conversation, or immediately after making love with him. Both of these activities increase serotonin production.

An autoimmune profile showed excessive T-helper cells (which are warming) and depressed T-suppressor cells (which are cooling). Her neurotransmitter profile identified her as being extremely serotonin deficient.

Jay prescribed clonazepam (a GABA agonist) and magnesium, and put her on a cooling regimen similar to the one described in the 28-day program. Having learned about the psychoemotional factors that affect her immune system, Laurie greatly reduced the stress in her life and has reaped the benefits. She no longer feels as if her body is overheating, and she has much better control over her MS symptoms.

Rheumatoid Arthritis and Cooling Deficiency

Rheumatoid arthritis (RA) is an inflammatory disease caused by an inadequate cooling neurotransmitter system that can't balance an overexcited warming system. When that happens, the immune system attacks the patient's joints, destroying cartilage and bone, resulting in swelling, stiffness, pain, and partial or complete loss of function. RA can also affect other parts of the body, including the neck, eyes, and mouth. Unlike osteoarthritis, RA symptoms happen almost exclusively in the morning, when the warming neurotransmitters are becoming even more active, thus aggravating an already-existing cooling deficit.

Researchers are actively working on treatments for this disease. One approach that seems particularly promising is to block a chemical messenger (called the *p38 kinase enzyme*) that produces inflammatory proteins. Interfering with p38 kinase effectively cools off an overheated immune system.

As we've seen in this chapter, cooling deficiencies are implicated in a wide variety of conditions and ailments that run the gamut from the annoying to the life-threatening and affect your mind, body, and behavior. Although that information is great to have, it's not the only reason you bought this book. In chapter 7 we'll take your knowledge of cooling deficiencies to the next level and give you a 28-day program that will help you get your neurotransmitters back in balance. When you're done, you'll be less restless, more alert, better able to manage your moods and emotions, and more in control of your weight. Many of the chronic symptoms that have plagued you for years will start to disappear. Life will be a lot more pleasant and you'll feel healthier and more comfortable.

CHAPTER 5

Are You Too Cool *and* Too Warm?

How Dual Warming and Cooling Deficiencies Affect Your Mind and Body

Michelle was one of Chris's most interesting patients, one whose symptoms were attributable to constantly flip-flopping warming and cooling neurotransmitter deficits.

A forty-one-year-old buyer for an exclusive chain of women's clothing boutiques, she was petite and extremely attractive but spoke in a high-pitched, squeaky voice that was at times too soft to hear. She appeared flighty and forgetful and began crying during her initial visit. She told Chris that she had been sexually abused as a child, which probably made her cooling deficient for most of her life. (Abused or battered people are generally serotonin deficient because of the lingering insecurity that abuse leaves them with.)

She married a powerful and successful fashion industry executive who had a dominant personality. Being with him and having plenty of money initially helped her feel safe, which raised her serotonin levels. But Michelle's husband was a very difficult man to please, and the harder she tried, the more dissatisfied he became. Michelle wanted to see a marriage counselor, but her husband refused, telling her it was a sign of weakness. This left her feeling hopelessly trapped, a situation that caused her chronic, unrelenting stress. She began feeling tired all the time and developed a variety of aches and pains.

She saw several doctors, who diagnosed her with a variety of infectious diseases and acute and chronic illnesses, and treated her with various courses of antibiotics. Judging from Michelle's history of neurotransmitter imbalance, Chris felt that she had been misdiagnosed—and given the wrong treatments. He felt that she didn't have any infections at all, but rather a chronic inflammation that was the result of a cooling (serotonin) deficiency so severe that it resulted in a relative warming (dopamine) excess. This kind of inflammation may sound, seem, and look like an infection, but it doesn't cause a fever the way a true infection would.

The years of dopamine excess put a tremendous stress on Michelle's body and caused her to look and feel older than she was. Eventually her dopamine system was no longer able to sustain the demand and burned itself out. That created an immediate dopamine deficiency, which resulted in chronic fatigue and the constant pain of fibromyalgia.

Michelle had been an avid runner, logging an hour or two a day for years. But for over a year and a half, she spent most of her days in bed, too depressed, tired, and pain ridden to get out, a fact she was able to keep from her husband for a while because she was out of work. When he eventually found out that she was unable to meet his demands as a wife, the two separated. Initially that made her depression worse. She saw a psychiatrist, who put her on Celexa, a serotonin-enhancing antidepressant that made her feel better. Increasing serotonin "healed" her brain enough to enable it to resume production of dopamine, which helped resolve her warming deficiency. But it didn't do much for her fatigue and muscle pain.

When she first came to see Chris she was taking 60 mg/day of Celexa, Valium for muscle relaxation, and Vicodin for pain. The combination of the three was contributing to her fatigue by increasing her cooling neurotransmitters, serotonin and GABA—but only for a short while. That also kept her from enjoying her freedom from the pressures of her marriage and the financial security her divorce settlement brought her. In a drug-induced stupor, she slept soundly but woke up feeling foggy and had a terrible time functioning during the day.

Michelle's twin deficiencies made her treatment somewhat complex. Increasing one neurotransmitter too much or too quickly might inadvertently drive the other down, further aggravating her imbalance. So Chris started Michelle on a diet high in complex carbohydrates, lean protein, and healthy fats to gently raise both her warming and cooling neurotransmitters at the same time. He also put her on the 28-day exercise rebuilding program described in chapter 8 that was designed to increase her ability to exercise without triggering any neurochemical imbalances or unwanted immune system activity.

After a week on this program, Michelle was feeling so much better that she went beyond the prescribed exercise limit, pushing herself beyond her tolerance. After three days of flulike symptoms she started the program again, this time sticking with it as prescribed.

Chris also weaned Michelle off her Valium and Vicodin and the multitude of herbs and supplements she was taking—slowly, to avoid the rebound seizures that sometimes occur when stopping Valium— and prescribed a mild sedative to have on hand as a last resort. He asked her to take 200 mg of tryptophan at bedtime along with 400 mg of magnesium to help her get to sleep without the heavy sedation. He also switched her from Celexa to Zoloft, an SSRI that helps maintain normal dopamine and serotonin levels.

Since starting her program, Michelle has adjusted well to her life circumstances. She's changed jobs, has begun having psychologically constructive relationships, and has resumed her former level of exercise and activity. She also took years off her physical appearance. This was partly a side effect of taking more interest in her appearance, but it was mainly the result of restoring her natural neurotransmitter balance.

How Does Dual Deficiency Work?

Very few things in life are completely black or white, and the same applies to neurotransmitter imbalances. Although many people reading this book will be able to define themselves in terms of a deficiency of either warming or cooling neurotransmitters, a sizable number will have deficiencies of both.

At this point you might reasonably ask how dual deficiency works—after all, both ends of a seesaw can't be down at the same time, right? When it comes to seesaws, that's true, but neurotransmitters often behave a little more subtly. Before we go on, let's do a quick review of the most common emotional and physical symptoms that are caused by either warming or cooling neurotransmitter deficiencies.

Warming Deficiency

Emotional Symptoms	Physical Symptoms
Denial	Low blood pressure
Depression	Fainting
Anger at oneself	Diminished body movement
Apathy	Parkinson's disease
Decreased arousal	Dry skin
Sexual disinterest or impotence	Cold intolerance
Brain fog	Weight gain and obesity
Inattentiveness	Diabetes
Impulsivity	Frequent, recurrent infections
Scattered thoughts	Predisposition to cancer
Low energy	Addictions
Lack of initiative or desire	
Frequent cravings for stimulants (particularly chocolate or caffeine)	

Cooling Deficiency

Emotional Symptoms	Physical Symptoms
Anger at others	Hypertension
Restlessness	Rapid heartbeat
Fear	Angina, heart disease
Withdrawal	Body jerks and twitches
Avoidant personality	Nausea
Being tearful	Sweating
Being hyperemotional	Heat intolerance
Hypersensitivity	Headaches
Being inhibited and shy	Chronic pain syndromes

(continued)

Obsessive behavior	Frequent allergies
Being prone to worry	Swelling or edema
Anxiety	Breast tenderness
Panic attacks	Predisposition to autoimmune diseases (such as rheumatoid arthritis and lupus)
Low self-esteem	
Craving carbohydrates	Sleep problems

A person with a dual NT deficiency could easily have symptoms from both charts, even though the underlying causes of the symptoms are contradictory. In psychiatry, having two or more conditions with different origins is called *comorbidity*. In our practices we see patients with a wide variety of comorbid conditions, including bipolar disease, autism, and treatment-resistant depression, that are related to dual-neurotransmitter deficits. Here are the most common combinations:

- low energy (low dopamine) and restlessness (low serotonin)
- depression (low dopamine) and anxiety (low serotonin)
- lack of mental sharpness (low dopamine) combined with obsessions and worry (low serotonin)
- fatigue (low dopamine) and muscle pain (low serotonin)
- craving for cigarettes and caffeine (low dopamine) as well as alcohol or tranquilizers (low serotonin)
- anger at oneself (low dopamine) and anger at others (low serotonin)
- diabetes (low dopamine) and heart problems (low serotonin)
- ADHD (low dopamine) and obsessive-compulsive disorder (low serotonin)

Stress and Dual Deficiency

Tens of thousands of years ago, when life was simpler, the brain could react to internal and external inputs and ensure *homeostasis*—the dynamic balance of dopamine and serotonin and the systems they control. Fabrics and foods were all natural, and stress consisted mostly of being chased by our numerous predators. There were no cell phones, no pagers, no laptops, no credit card bills, no alarm clocks, no carpools, no jet lag, no exhaust fumes or cigarette smoke to pollute the air, no hazardous chemicals in the water, and no processed or fast foods (except for animals that were too slow to get away from the primitive hunter-gatherer).

Today life is quite different. But unfortunately, as marvelous as the human brain is, it hasn't been able to evolve quickly enough to keep up with changes in lifestyle, diet, stress levels, noise, and food. Chemically and physiologically speaking, we're built to deal with life the way it was 10,000 years ago. Constantly bombarded with modern-day environmental, chemical, sensory, nutritional, financial, and social stressors, our brain is easily overwhelmed, and warming or cooling neurotransmitter deficits develop. When those stressors last long enough (which they frequently do), the result is often a deficit of *both* neurotransmitter groups.

One of the major culprits in creating dual deficits is the warming stress hormone cortisol. We know from extensive animal and human studies that prolonged stress elevates blood levels of cortisol. This has three effects on our neurotransmitter balance:

1. The brain releases serotonin in an attempt to offset the heating influence of cortisol. But if levels of cortisol remain elevated, the serotonin system gets overloaded, resulting in a kind of burnout.
2. Once cortisol has burned through the brain's serotonin capacity, it starts undermining dopamine, starving brain cells by interfering with the transport of glucose from the bloodstream.
3. At this point brain cells are unable to produce adequate amounts of either serotonin or dopamine. If this condition continues, brain cells begin to die, causing permanent brain damage.

Somewhere in the middle of this three-step process is what the National Institutes of Mental Health researcher Robert Post calls "kindling." Post's theory is that each exposure to stress increases the brain's sensitivity to the next exposure. In other words, the more you get stressed out, anxious, and depressed, the easier and more likely it becomes to get that way again—and the less it takes to trigger those reactions. It's as though the cells that have been inflamed once by stress put a match to their neighboring cells, gradually creating a bigger and bigger fire, in the way that small pieces of kindling ignite a large log that might not otherwise catch fire by itself.

Life's Ultimate On/Off Switches

Dopamine, serotonin, and the other neurotransmitters are both the message and the messenger, carrying instructions and triggering chemical reactions throughout our body and brain. But as powerful as they are, neurotransmitters can't penetrate the outer membrane of the cell. Instead, they deliver their message to receptors, which open up channels between the outside of the cell and the part of the cell that will generate the proper response.

These channels are called *intracellular transduction pathways* (ITPs), and the molecules that travel along them, carrying the neurotransmitters' messages, are called *protein kinases.* Protein kinases act as cellular switches, turning on the parts of the cell that are required for the response and turning off the rest.

BDNF

Perhaps the most important of these ITPs is a compound called *brain-derived neurotrophic factor* (BDNF). BDNF is associated with the production of new neurons and helping them survive. In addition, BDNF is the pathway that both dopamine and serotonin use to relay their message.

When BDNF levels are adequate, the kinases can do their job. Chemical messages get where they're supposed to go, cells grow and divide, and life goes on. The more BDNF inside a cell, the better messages can travel within it and the more effectively that cell can communicate with its neighbors. But when BDNF is depleted, the result is a dual NT deficiency, since neither dopamine nor serotonin can get their messages to their cellular targets. If the BDNF pathway isn't repaired quickly, cells start to die.

A number of factors are known to increase BDNF, which in turn reverses brain damage in the hippocampus. These include any kind of exercise, a number of supplements and herbs that we'll discuss in chapter 8, antidepressants—regardless of whether they boost serotonin or dopamine—and positive feelings associated with joy, community, companionship, and hope. Research into finding antidepressant drugs that work directly on BDNF instead of serotonin or dopamine is ongoing.

Conversely, prolonged stress, anxiety, and depression all elevate cortisol levels, which effectively shuts down BDNF. MRI scans of patients with these conditions have shown decreased volume in the hippocampus. Persistently elevated cortisol levels and disrupted BDNF have been associated with neurodegenerative diseases such as Alzheimer's and Parkinson's, and a number of other conditions such as Lou Gehrig's disease (ALS), stroke, spinal cord injury, and chronic alcohol use.

While we aren't saying that prolonged stress *causes* these devastating conditions, we are saying that it certainly contributes to them by making people more vulnerable. In fact, we believe that the majority of dual deficit conditions are either caused or severely aggravated by prolonged stress, elevated cortisol levels, and BDNF interference. These conditions can affect every aspect of your mind, body, and behavior. Let's take a look at some of them in greater detail.

Anxiety and Depression and Dual Deficiency

Over 19 million Americans suffer from diagnosed anxiety disorders, and about half of those have symptoms of depression at the same time. And of the 20 million or so Americans who suffer from depression, roughly two-thirds also have anxiety symptoms. Although anxiety and depression are frequent companions, there are significant differences between the two. On the most fundamental level, anxiety is an overwhelming feeling of helplessness, while depression is an overwhelming feeling of hopelessness.

Still, there's a growing feeling in the mental health community that anxiety and depression may actually be symptoms of a single underlying condition. The American Psychiatric Association (APA) is preliminarily referring to it as *mixed anxiety-depressive disorder.*

Take a moment to answer the following questions. Are you now experiencing or have you recently experienced:

- concentration or memory difficulties?
- sleep disturbances?
- fatigue or low energy?
- irritability?
- worry?
- being easily moved to tears?
- hypervigilance?
- anticipating the worst?

- hopelessness or pessimism about the future?
- low self-esteem or feelings of worthlessness?

According to the APA, if you answered yes to at least four of the above questions and if your symptoms have lasted for at least four weeks, you may have a mixed anxiety-depressive disorder.

Cyclothymia and Dual Deficiency

When the balance between warming and cooling states is disrupted, some people—such as those with mixed anxiety-depression disorder—experience deficits of both systems at the same time. Others switch back and forth from one deficit to the other. On any given day, people with an incredibly widespread but little-recognized condition called *cyclothymia* can vacillate between optimistic, high-dopamine states and pessimistic, low-serotonin states. Depending on the circumstances, they can go from being overly cautious, anxious, and sensitive to being aggressive, extroverted, and taking risks; from periods of depression, fatigue, increased need for sleep, and excessive eating to periods of high energy, nervousness, decreased need for sleep, and euphoric mood. Part of the reason that cyclothymia isn't diagnosed more often is that patients who suffer from it tend to seek out medical help only when they're feeling depressed; they rarely complain when they're feeling especially good.

If you think this sounds like bipolar disorder (what used to be called "manic depression"), you're absolutely right. In fact, cyclothymia, which literally means "circular spirit," is sometimes called *soft bipolar.* But the difference is one of degree. True bipolar disorders are marked by severe manic episodes that last for days or weeks at a time, alternating with severe, sometimes suicidal depressions lasting just as long. People with cyclothymia have much milder and much shorter "up" and "down" periods, but their constantly changing moods can still have a very negative impact on their work and social lives.

In people with bipolar disorder or cyclothymia, the balance between warming and cooling neurotransmitters is easily disrupted by small changes in the patient's physical or emotional environment. Sleep deprivation, jet lag, a change in season, weather, and menstrual cycles are all known triggers.

Irritable Bowel Syndrome (IBS) and Dual Deficiency

IBS is a common gastrointestinal disorder characterized by abdominal pain and alternating constipation and diarrhea. Between 50 and 90 percent of people with IBS experience anxiety, panic attacks, and depression. IBS is also frequently associated with migraine and PMS. Genetic studies have linked IBS with abnormalities of the serotonin system, and recent drugs for IBS interact with serotonin receptors in the gut. In addition, an imbalance of glutamate may be responsible for the heightened pain and sensitivity of IBS patients.

PMS and Dual Deficiency

As we discussed, PMS affects about 25 million women and can cause over 150 different symptoms. Some of those symptoms, such as depression, bloating, breast swelling and tenderness, and morning face puffiness, are associated with warming NT deficiencies. Others, such as depression, anxiety, irritability, and cravings for carbohydrates, are caused by cooling deficiencies. Women with dual NT deficits commonly complain of both kinds of symptoms.

Migraines and Dual Deficiency

Migraine headaches are caused by an instability in the membrane of brain cells. This instability causes sudden shifts in neurotransmitter levels in the brain, which overexcites the cells. It's also responsible for the auras many sufferers experience immediately prior to the onset of the headache. There's a 75 percent correlation between migraines and cyclothymia. And migraines are also associated with a number of other neurological and psychiatric conditions, including depression, anxiety, panic, and epilepsy.

ADD with OCD, Tourette's, Learning Disabilities, Anxiety, or Depression

Twenty-seven-year-old Jonathan was referred to Jay by a court-appointed attorney who was defending Jonathan on an indecent assault charge. Jonathan had been fired from numerous jobs for his rude, disrespectful behavior, and he seemed to pride himself on his ability to alienate, insult, intimidate, and hurt anyone who tried to befriend him. But what had gotten him arrested was having groped and licked a female ticket taker at a movie theater.

Sitting in Jay's waiting room he was sullen and rude. Physically, he was obese. At first, Jonathan denied that he had any kind of problem at all. But he acknowledged that he was sometimes impulsive, and added that he also suffered from recurring headaches and insomnia. After a lot of cajoling from the attorney, Jonathan agreed to allow Jay to do a neurotransmitter profile, which revealed extreme deficiencies of both serotonin and dopamine. The combination was responsible for Jonathan's "emotional Tourette's syndrome," his aggressive, sometimes violent behavior, his inability to inhibit negative behavior, and his seeming disregard for the consequences of his actions.

Jonathan had seen numerous specialists and mental health professionals, and the list of medications he'd taken over the years was a page and a half long. However, most of them had triggered adverse or paradoxical (the opposite of what would normally be expected) reactions, and Jonathan had been declared a "treatment failure."

In reviewing Jonathan's medical history, Jay found out that Jonathan had had similar problems ever since he was a boy—severe mood swings, throwing things such as knives at his teachers and his parents, and even killing a neighbor's rabbit. Despite a genius-level IQ, he'd been thrown out of several high schools and had never attended college.

Because of the severity of Jonathan's problems, Jay immediately put him on Abilify, a promising new drug approved for the treatment of psychosis. Abilify works like a neurochemical thermostat, speeding up the production of warming neurotransmitters if the brain seems dominated by cooling, and increasing the production of cooling NTs if the brain seems overheated.

Within a week on Abilify, Jonathan had experienced what he called "a complete personality change." He was calm, focused, articulate, and polite. He even expressed regret for his past inappropriate behavior and described feeling like a bird let out of its cage. Able to express empathy, he hugged his mother for the first time in several years and expressed a desire to enroll in college.

Although attention deficit disorder is a classic dopamine deficiency, it is frequently seen in combination with cooling deficiency (or warming excess) conditions such as obsessive-compulsive disorder, Tourette's, anxiety, mood swings, rage, and depression. In addition, about 30 percent of people with ADD have or will develop bipolar disorder (compared to only 2 percent of people without ADD), and about 16 percent of people with OCD already have cyclothymia, which increases their chances of developing bipolar disorder later on. People with either of these combined conditions are at especially high risk of developing other psychological problems as well.

To treat ADD by itself, physicians frequently prescribe dopamine agonists such as Ritalin or Adderall. But when ADD is combined with one or more of the above conditions, dopamine agonists alone often aggravate symptoms of the associated conditions. Bipolar disorder, for example, is caused by excessively high levels of the warming NT glutamate. Dopamine-stimulating drugs increase glutamate levels even further and can precipitate manic attacks.

Adding cooling antioxidants (such as omega-3 fatty acids) or cooling GABA agonists (such as lithium, Neurontin, or Depakote) to the cocktail is extremely effective.

William's Story:
Dual Deficiency and Adult ADHD

William grew up in an affluent suburb of New York, went to the best private schools, and summered on Martha's Vineyard. He started getting into trouble with the law at twelve, getting arrested for breaking store windows and shoplifting. At fourteen, he developed a crack habit and would take the subway to one of the roughest neighborhoods in the South Bronx to score. Within a year of getting his driver's license, he'd been pulled over four times for driving under the influence. He picked up prostitutes and did IV drugs. There was something about danger and living on the edge that excited him. But when he woke up from three months in a coma after driving his father's $150,000 Porsche into a tree, he realized that something needed to change.

On his first visit to Jay, William underwent a series of tests, and two things were clear. First, he was incredibly lucky that he was HIV negative. Second, his warming neurotransmitter profile was so low that they were barely detectable. Reviewing his childhood history, it became evident that William expressed symptoms of ADHD even as a toddler. He was aggressive toward other children, oppositional, and impulsive. Although he was highly intelligent, he was easily bored and barely passed through school. He began smoking at fourteen. William's history of dangerous, excessive, self-destructive behavior was the result of his brain's attempts to feel better by stimulating its reward centers.

When a diagnosis of adult ADHD was established, Jay prescribed Adderall, a dopamine-enhancing medication. The results were almost immediate. William felt calmer, he was able to focus, and his urges to take illicit drugs and drive excessively fast almost disappeared. At the same time, though, another problem developed.

William had apparently always been slightly obsessive-compulsive, a problem that was overshadowed by his warming-deficit condition. He'd get an idea into his head that he absolutely had to have something—perhaps a new car or an expensive stereo—and he would be obsessed with the object until he got it. Although raising William's dopamine levels reduced his self-destructive behavior, it made his obsessions a lot worse. Jay added a low dose of Lexapro, an SSRI, and the combination did the trick, increasing his warming neurotransmitters enough to reduce the dangerous behavior and addiction, and increasing the cooling neurotransmitters just enough to eliminate the obsessions.

Other Physical Problems Related to Dual Deficiencies

Dual neurotransmitter deficits, particularly the potent combination of depression and anxiety, have been linked with a number of other conditions, including ulcers, angina, diabetes, glucose control, thyroid disorders, poor immune system function, and heart problems.

Parkinson's and Alzheimer's and Dual Deficiency

Parkinson's disease is marked by the death of dopamine-producing cells in the brain, and dopamine-stimulating drugs are the treatment of choice. The problem is that increasing warming also increases the production of free radicals, which creates oxidative stress and overheats the brain. Adding antioxidants to the dopamine agonists for treatment of Parkinson's may protect the brain against the excessive free radical production that is so strongly associated with increasing warming neurotransmitters.

Alzheimer's disease is generally thought to be caused by a deficit of the warming neurotransmitter acetylcholine. As with Parkinson's, stimulating acetylcholine often simultaneously increases the production of another warming NT, glutamate. Overly high levels of glutamate (or excessively low levels of glutamate's opposite, GABA), are linked to brain cell death. Combining traditional acetylcholine agonists with Memantine, a glutamate blocker now in clinical trials, may help prevent the progression of Alzheimer's.

Sandy's Story: Dual Deficiencies, Cancer, and Anxiety

Chris saw Sandy a week after she was diagnosed with localized breast cancer. Ironically, she had made the appointment to see him for an evaluation and for a program to prevent disease one month before. At the time she made her appointment, Chris suggested she see her gynecologist and have a mammogram before arriving so they could review the data together. At their initial meeting they discussed the options for treating her cancer. Because he's not an oncologist, Chris recommended that she see one. She did, and she underwent a lumpectomy and radiation without chemotherapy. A few months later, Sandy returned to see Chris to discuss her problem and her feelings.

A forty-four-year-old cosmetics salesperson, Sandy seemed to have it all together. She was neat, well organized, and engaging, and looked ten years younger than she was. She exercised three times a week for at least an hour, slept well, and ate a low-calorie diet to maintain her weight and figure. But on the inside, she felt like she was going to explode and reported feeling "uptight" and "fidgety." Chris told her the anxiety was normal for a person dealing with the shock and trauma of cancer. He suggested she focus on how fortunate she was to have had an early diagnosis, not how frightening it was to have the disease. He suggested she begin a program of brain balancing to help get hold of her emotions and redirect her anxiousness and restlessness toward helping herself grow healthier and finding ways to help others.

Cancer is often associated with low warming neurotransmitter levels, and in doing some additional testing, Chris discovered that Sandy's thyroid levels were baseline and her testosterone levels were low. (Although testosterone is generally considered a "male" hormone, women need minimum levels to maintain optimal health, in the same way that men need minimum amounts of estrogen, the "female" hormone.)

But Sandy was restless and anxious, two classic symptoms of low cooling neurotransmitters. Sandy was deficient in both warming and cooling neurotransmitters. Following the rules that grew out of his and Jay's work and experience, Chris started Sandy on the program described in chapter 8 to deal with her cooling deficiency first. This included supplementation with 5-HTP, the amino acid inositol, and a B-complex vitamin with B-6 and folic acid, aromatherapy, and yoga.

After a few months she was no longer feeling nervous, and was ready to focus on rebalancing her warming neurotransmitters, which would help her immune system fight her cancer. Chris gradually shifted Sandy from the cooling-deficiency program to the warming-deficiency program.

Cancer and anxiety are both complex disorders. Although it's clear that diet, sedentary activity, sleep deprivation, and stress related to self-perspective contribute to cancer and play an important role in survival, these factors are not the sole cause. Just as there are many contributors to cancer, so too are there many factors that result in anxiety. Recognizing the role that neurotransmitter imbalances play in each problem and correcting them through an individualized, progressive program can help a person with health challenges such as Sandy's cope and overcome both. Sandy believes she was lucky to have had and survived cancer with as little trauma and emotional distress as she did, and she credits part of her success to making changes in her life.

In this chapter we've discussed the specific symptoms and conditions that are caused or aggravated by simultaneous deficiencies of both warming and cooling neurotransmitters. In chapter 8 you'll find a 28-day plan that's designed to help you heal your dual deficiency, restore proper balance, and create a new healthier you. If you haven't already done so, we strongly encourage you to take some time *before* implementing the plan to read chapters 3 and 4, which explore in greater detail the specific issues associated with each type of deficiency. If you want to skip those chapters and get started right away, just be sure to come back and read them before the end of the twenty-eight days. Whenever you start, you'll be well on your way to enjoying the increased energy, better mood, reduced cravings, and other benefits you'll get from balancing your levels.

PART TWO

The Balance Your Brain, Balance Your Life 28-Day Programs

CHAPTER 6

Warming Up

How to Balance Your Warming Neurotransmitter Deficiency

Our physical, mental, emotional, and immune systems, as well as others, are linked at the most basic levels and work together to create a fully integrated system: us. When something changes in any part of our body, something will change in the mind as well. And if we change something in our brain, a change will happen somewhere else in the body.

If you're reading this, it may be because the warming mechanisms that your brain and body use to reward you, give you pleasure, and make you feel good aren't working quite as well as they should. This may have made you feel fatigued, weighed-down, or depressed, and may be responsible for some of the habits that have made you feel worse.

That's why we've put together the comprehensive 28-day Warming Program, which will enable you to recover from the tiredness, food cravings, weight problems, lack of motivation, mental fog, and other symptoms that have plagued you.

You'll find it easy to increase your warming neurotransmitter levels, and once you start the program you'll begin seeing some changes almost immediately: You'll be more alert, have better concentration, and feel better.

We ask you to stick with the program for at least twenty-eight days. Why twenty-eight? Well, there are some very lucky (and very rare) people who will be able to correct their imbalance immediately. However, for the overwhelming majority of us, the path is much longer. Practice doesn't make perfect; it makes permanent. But a habit, whether good or bad, doesn't become part of the fabric of your being until you do it many times. After years of experience, we've seen that a month is a reasonable amount of time to start the process. After twenty-eight days on the program, your new, healthier habits may not yet be permanent, but you'll be well on your way. The changes may be subtle at first, but within a few weeks, they'll be recognizable not only to you, but to everyone around you as well.

Our self-care program has seven basic parts. These steps include lifestyle changes, dietary modification, physical exercise, specific herbal and vitamin remedies, and even hormonal and pharmacological approaches if necessary. Here's a brief overview:

1. *Perspective and worldview.* The first step in implementing this program is to change your thinking. Learning to believe in yourself and in your worth as a person is critical to achieving mind and body health.
2. *Lifestyle.* Changing your lifestyle—your hobbies, activities, habits, and the environment you live and work in—is one of the most effective ways to boost your warming neurotransmitter levels. It's also one of the hardest, because you may have to overcome years of bad habits. The trick is to try to remember the things that make you happy and incorporate as many of them into your daily routine as possible. The more dopamine-, norepinephrine-, and acetylcholine-raising activities you do, the better off you'll be.
3. *Diet and supplements.* A warming deficiency is, by definition, a cooling excess, which is a low-energy state. The basic diet is high in protein, with frequent meals to help sustain energy production. Keep carbohydrates to a minimum during the day, except for the low-energy period between 3:00 P.M. and 5:00 P.M. You may need to bring back some carbs at night, depending on factors such as your body composition, activity level, disease predispositions, and sleep problems.
4. *Exercise and activity.* This exercise program addresses the specific needs of people with warming NT deficits. Warming-deficient people often get so excited by the progress they're making that they overdo

it and burn out too quickly. For that reason our program is designed to ease you in gradually, allowing your brain to safely step up warming neurotransmitter production without overloading itself.

5. *Sleep.* How long and how well you sleep is, in a way, a reflection of the success or failure of all the steps that have come before. Ideally you should be able to get at least seven—but no more than eight—uninterrupted hours of restful sleep every night.

6. *Maintenance.* Once you've raised your warming neurotransmitters enough to get your mind and body back in balance, you need to keep them there. We'll show you how to maintain your disposition and keep yourself from falling into a deficiency state again.

7. *Working with your doctor.* If you've made a serious effort to stay on the program for twenty-eight days and you still aren't feeling well, make an appointment to see your doctor. He or she may be able to offer some more advanced testing to pinpoint your deficiency and may be able to prescribe hormones and/or medications. Even if you do end up going this route, we strongly urge you to stay on the program. It provides a solid base that will improve the effectiveness of any drug or hormone therapy your doctor may prescribe.

Do Things Early in the Day

There's an ancient Ayurvedic saying that all intelligence awakes with the morning. But intelligence isn't all that rises along with the sun. Your warming neurotransmitter levels ebb and flow throughout the day, and they're at their peak in the morning. So take advantage of that extra boost and do as many warming-NT-increasing activities as you can before lunch. If you wait too long, your warming levels will drop, and you may lose the energy and motivation to do the things you need to be doing. Generally speaking, you want to increase stimulation during the day and decrease it at night so you can properly recover from your daytime activities.

Of course, you can't do everything in the morning. Because you need to eat throughout the day, the diet and nutrition section of our plan will tell you what you need to do to get you through the afternoon and evening warming NT lulls. And, hopefully, you'll be doing most of your sleeping at night. But try to implement the perspective, lifestyle, and exercise parts of the program in the morning. Doing so will make it easier for your brain to reshape and recondition itself.

Getting Under Way

None of the steps we're suggesting, whether they involve lifestyle, amino acids, herbs, and/or vitamins, will interact negatively with one another and none will be contradictory or cancel each other out. However, we recommend that you check with your personal physician before you start this program. We also strongly recommend that you don't take any prescription medication or hormones that you read about in this book—and especially don't combine them—except as directed by your physician.

Resist the urge to jump ahead or to skip days, and pay close attention to how you feel as you're going through the program. If you find yourself feeling sick, agitated, frustrated, angry, or giddy, take a day or two off and start the program again. If you continue to feel bad, see your doctor.

Before you actually start the program, we want you to have a firm understanding of what you're going to be doing and why. Here's a detailed look at each of the steps.

Perspective and Worldview

The most common cause of warming deficiencies is emotional pain, which can arise from a number of different sources. These include low self-esteem, unresolved conflict and anger, loss of something you value, or the anticipation of that loss. If these or any other similar sources of emotional pain influence your thoughts and feelings, they're playing a role in your warming deficiency.

Warming-deficient people tend toward depression. This could be the result of genetics, conscious or unconscious unresolved conflicts, the day-to-day levels of stress in your life, or some combination of those factors. Whatever the cause, it's exaggerated by a lack of worldview, by not having a firm idea of why you are here and what you would like to be and do. You don't have to have all the answers, but having a sense of purpose in life can be very helpful in maintaining balance, especially in difficult times.

Increasing Your Enjoyment

As a warming-deficient person, you also need to learn to find sources of enjoyment, pleasure, and motivation. This does *not* have to be some kind of spiritual or religious quest, although if thinking in those terms helps you, that's what you should be doing. Ask yourself the following questions:

1. What do I really like in life and what do I most enjoy doing?
2. Whom do I enjoy being with and having around to do these things with?
3. What have I done in my life that gave me the greatest joy?
4. What are my favorite colors, fragrances, sights, and textures?
5. Where do I like spending my time?
6. If I could live anywhere and do anything, where would that be and what would I do?

Your answers to these questions will get you back in touch with some of the things that have made your life more enjoyable in the past and have given you the energy to move forward. You don't have to think about them all the time, only when you need a little boost. If you can focus your mind on at least one positive memory when you're feeling particularly unmotivated or depressed, you'll be taking an important step in accomplishing your goals.

If you find it hard to answer these questions, discuss them with a friend or someone you trust. Often just talking about the things that evade you will help make them clear. Talking to someone who is trained to listen and offer insight can be valuable, but it isn't always necessary. A spouse, friend, cleric, or other confidant acting in the role of a supportive listener can be equally effective, more convenient, and less expensive. Try them first. To make this work, you must inform the listener you are not asking him or her for the answer, but rather looking for it within yourself. If you try and don't quite get there, or the listener can't resist telling you how to live or what you have to do to solve your problems, look to a professional.

A counselor must be a good fit and meet your individual needs. You should feel comfortable working together and always try more than one before you make your final decision (in other words, interview prospective counselors before committing to a series of appointments). And if things don't seem like they're going well after a few sessions, don't be shy about making a change. This is one area of your life that really is all about you.

If You Are Warming Deficient with Low Self-Esteem

You need to balance your view of yourself and your accomplishments. Begin by acknowledging that you have done a lot of good for people in your lifetime. Accept yourself and move on. All love, kindness, and generosity are derived from self-love and self-acceptance. Optimal health cannot be achieved without it. Do the things you like to do each day until they become your routine. Develop a system to help minimize doubt, self-criticism, and distress as soon as you recognize feeling them. The system itself doesn't matter, as long as you make it part of your daily life. Try breathing deeply as many times a day as you can and for as many breaths as you can stand. Breathing deeply with long exhalations ignites the production of warming NTs and cools the brain, allowing for greater warming with the next breath. Progressive relaxation, meditation, and cognitive reinforcement are also excellent choices.

Address the spiritual aspect of your thoughts—not necessarily with religious principles or pursuits, but with your own system of beliefs. Forgive yourself and others. Remain open and curious. Acknowledge your goodness and recognize the good things you do for others. But don't look to them for your satisfaction; give it to yourself. Finally, use the power and experience of love to raise your awareness of the abundant things in your life. You are rich in the things that money cannot buy, as well as the things it can. Be good to yourself and allow that to quiet the voice of inner doubt and dissatisfaction.

Each week of the program will have a different theme, and for each day we'll give you a specific mission statement to focus on that will reinforce that theme. Here are several ways you can increase the effectiveness of these mission statements:

- Set aside at least fifteen minutes every day when you can be quiet and alone. Repeat the statement to yourself several times. Think about it but don't judge it. Add images and visualize what you're saying.
- At night, just before bed, write out the next day's statement and tape it up in places you're likely to go the next morning, such as the bathroom mirror or the refrigerator.

- Make each statement your computer's screen saver for the day.
- Write the statement out ten times, but from several different perspectives: "I am healthy." "She, Jane, is healthy." "You are healthy."

Lifestyle

Even before you start the 28-day Warming Program, the first thing to do is take two minutes—that's all you'll need—to jot down a list of ten things that give you enjoyment and pleasure. No, don't do it later. Grab a pen and do it now. Part of your problem is getting the motivation to follow through with things that are good for you. "I think I'll wait" is the epitaph of the warming-deficient person. To make it a little easier for you, we've even left you some blank lines.

1. _____

2. _____

3. _____

4. _____

5. _____

6. _____

7. _____

8. _____

9. _____

10. _____

Okay, now go back to your list and put a check mark next to the items that you actually do on a regular basis. Of those, put an H next to the ones that are healthy and pleasurable, and a U next to the ones that are unhealthy.

There's probably not a lot of overlap between the items that you do regularly and the healthy items. The place to start is by doing more things that you like to do and that you know are good for you. You can do that very easily by making a few simple lifestyle changes. We'll give you some specific suggestions every day in the 28-day program that follows. But feel free to add as many of the items from your list as you'd like. When it comes to increasing your warming neurotransmitters, the more lifestyle changes you make, the better.

Specific Recommendations to a Warming-Deficient Patient with ADD/ADHD

A day doesn't go by that we don't see someone who either has ADD or has a child affected by it. And most of them have grasped for miracle cures in books or on the Internet. Unfortunately, there aren't any.

ADD and ADHD manifest themselves in many different ways and cause many different symptoms, including problems with attentiveness, cognition, distractibility, organization, impulsivity, hyperactivity, inability to focus, interpersonal relationships, and a tendency toward drug abuse. If you have ADD or ADHD, take an honest look at how your condition affects your life. If any of the cognitive, social, or behavioral symptoms are truly diminishing the quality of your life, speak with a qualified professional about appropriate medication. In our practices, we've had tremendous success with stimulants, Wellbutrin, Provigil, and Straterra. And despite the prevailing wisdom that these drugs cause other problems, such as drug addiction later in life, we've found that the exact opposite is true.

If your symptoms are annoying but not significantly hurting your quality of life, we suggest that you implement as many of the elements of this 28-day plan as you can. Ideally, you should start with the perspective and worldview sections, but you may need to start with some nutritional supplement or prescription remedies first in order to give you the focus and attention you'll need to stay on course with the rest of the program. Diet has proven very important to adults and children suffering from ADD and/or ADHD.

Diet

As a warming-deficient person, the cornerstone of your diet is to reduce the amount of calories you consume. As we explained earlier, there's a direct relationship between warming neurotransmitter deficiency and a condition called *insulin resistance syndrome* (IRS).

The average North American diet is especially high in calories and saturated fat. These harmful foods act in the brain like drugs, triggering cravings and ultimately depleting warming neurotransmitter levels, particularly dopamine. As you reduce your calories, several things happen simultaneously. First, your cells will gradually become more receptive to insulin. This means that instead of converting the calories you eat into fat, your cells will be able to burn them for energy. You'll lose weight—especially around your middle. Second, reducing calories will restore the production of dopamine and other warming neurotransmitters in your brain. Third, you'll reduce cravings and rebound eating.

Reducing your caloric intake will also have a dramatically positive effect on your immune system. As you age, your immune system becomes less sensitive and less responsive. This is true for everyone but especially for people with warming deficiencies, whose neurotransmitter imbalance puts them at particularly high risk for cancer and infection. The reason for this increased vulnerability is that the warming deficiency reduces the size and function of an organ called the *thymus,* which produces cancer-fighting *T-cells.* And as if that weren't bad enough, as we age, our T-cells become less responsive to the signals that normally stimulate them to fight infection and cancer. This situation is exaggerated in warming-deficient people. But reducing calories reverses the shrinking of the thymus and recharges our T-cells, making them more alert and responsive to any alien invaders.

The most important thing you can do to reduce calories is to revise the composition of your diet. A good dopamine- and norepinephrine-enhancing diet will include about 40 percent lean protein, 30 percent carbohydrates from vegetables and starches, and 30 percent healthy fats such as nuts, olives, and soy products. The more protein you eat, the more dopamine your brain will release. This doesn't mean, of course, that you should eat nothing but protein. Doing so would only replace one imbalance and set of problems with a different one. As a general guide, think of things this way: proteins wake you up, starches put you to sleep, and fats make either effect last longer.

If You Are Overweight or Obese and Warming Deficient

Permanent weight control requires making permanent changes in your life. It starts with changing the way you think—about yourself, your world, and everyone and everything in it.

- Eat mindfully. Pay attention to what you eat, when you eat it, what you're thinking just before you eat, and how the food you eat makes you feel. Many people eat for reasons that have nothing to do with hunger: boredom, depression, anger, frustration, and so on. Figuring out why you do what you do is the first step to being able to break the pattern.
- Avoid fad diets. Every week there's a new plan that "guarantees" that it will help you lose all the weight you want. But these diets almost never deliver the goods.
- Take green tea extract and fish oil supplements. Hardly a fad, green tea has been used by doctors for thousands of years. The active ingredient of green tea raises norepinephrine levels, which stimulates metabolism, causing more fat burning. Several preliminary studies have shown that overweight people lost as much as 5 percent of their body weight after taking green tea extract for three months. As for fish oil, it significantly lowers triglycerides and acts as a natural insulin sensitizing agent, which reduces the chance that you'll develop insulin resistance syndrome.

Protein

You'll begin changing the composition of your diet by increasing the amount of protein you eat every day. This won't *directly* increase your warming neurotransmitter levels, but the net result is the same. Amino acids create proteins, including tyrosine (which is what dopamine and norepinephrine are made from), choline (which is a precursor to acetylcholine), and L-glutamine (which is one of the precursors of glutamate). By increasing your protein intake you'll be providing your system with the means to produce more of the neurotransmitters you need. Of course, you'll need to be selective about the kind of protein you eat. We recommend that you get your protein from whey and egg whites or from lean meats (red or white), such as poultry (turkey, quail, pheasant, free-range, no hormone is best) and fish. Don't be afraid to try new things in your efforts to overcome your deficiency. If you're a meat eater, for example, you'll find that well-prepared antelope, elk, venison, and other game meats are just as appetizing as any domesticated meat. Plus, they have the distinct advantage of almost always being hormone- and pesticide-free.

Carbohydrates

Your second step is to look at your intake of carbohydrates and fats. Carbohydrates are a vital part of a healthy diet and are a major source of energy. The potential problem is the connection between carbohydrates and insulin levels in your brain. Eating a high-carbohydrate (or high-sugar) diet raises insulin levels, which eventually leads to insulin resistance and all its negative side effects. Your metabolism, which is your ability to burn calories, slows and you end up gaining weight.

We suggest that you limit your carbohydrate intake to complex carbohydrates. Have vegetable carbs (including green leafy and other colorful vegetables, legumes of all kinds) in the morning. Eat starchy vegetables such as tubers (carrots and other root vegetables) with your evening meal to help you relax at the end of the day. Allow yourself a serving or two of potatoes, rice, or pasta if you like. Try to avoid bread during the 28-day plan, since bread is a concentrated form of starch that is too easy to overeat. Avoiding bread makes lowering your starch intake a lot easier.

Fats

The connection between dopamine and fats is equally important. A large percentage of brain receptors are made from fats, and the amount of fat in your diet has a direct impact on the responsiveness of those receptors. But be careful: all fats are not created equal. We strongly recommend that you stay as far away from saturated fats and *trans fatty acids* (also called partially hydrogenated oils) as you possibly can. These foods have no place in a healthy diet. They can reduce blood circulation by causing blood cells to clump together. They also keep the brain from properly synthesizing dopamine and norepinephrine, which are responsible for mental energy and clear thinking. Not surprisingly, this leads to fatigue and sluggish thinking. In the presence of norepinephrine (which you're increasing by eating more protein), saturated fats become unstable, causing a condition called *oxidative stress,* which in turn produces the free radicals responsible for causing tissue and organ damage. The higher the level of saturated fats and trans fats, the less the brain responds to warming NTs.

On the other hand, polyunsaturated fats—such as nuts and nut oils, monounsaturated fats like olive and canola oils, soy products including soy butter, and the famous omega-3 and omega-6 fatty acids that come from cold-water fish—are exactly what you need. Omega-3 fatty acids promote better neurotransmission of the warming NTs. Recent research from France showed that animals with high levels of fatty acids had high levels of dopamine in the brain. Conversely, deficiencies of essential fatty acids (omega-3 and omega-6) were linked to deficiencies of dopamine and loss of function in the areas of the brain involved in mood and learning. Other studies have found that high levels of fatty acids don't actually increase dopamine levels. Instead, they simply make dopamine receptors more sensitive—the overall levels may not change, but the brain becomes more responsive to what's there. The result is the same: an increase in the dopamine effect.

A high intake of saturated fat and cholesterol has been shown to double the risk of dementia. In contrast, increasing fish consumption, predominantly cold-water fish, leads to a 70 percent reduction in the risk of dementia. Researchers are now investigating the effectiveness of fatty acid supplements such as the omega-3 and omega-6 capsules in treating depression. Stay tuned.

The best sources of essential fatty acids are supplements, walnut oil, canola, and especially olive oil. Fish are also an excellent source, but watch out for king mackerel, swordfish, and tilefish, all of which are high in mercury.

Treating neurotransmitter deficiencies requires a strict elimination of foods that are commonly known to be allergenic. These include wheat, dairy, corn, soy, and peanuts. Raw food diets and diets devoid of processed flavor and white sugar also have their place. However, they are often impractical, and sometimes the stress involved in sticking to that kind of diet outweighs the benefit.

With the assistance of our colleague, nutritionist Carl Germano, RD, CNS, CDN, we've included a complete 28-day meal plan as part of the Warming Program. The diet in this chapter provides 1,700 calories per day. However, your caloric requirements may be somewhat different. To determine how many calories you need, do one of the following:

1. If you're a woman, multiply your weight in pounds by 12 if you're inactive, 13 if you do light work or exercise, 14 if you do light or moderate work or exercise, 15 for moderate to heavy work or exercise, and 16 for heavy work or exercise.
2. If you are a man, multiply your weight in pounds by 13 if you're inactive, 14 for light work or exercise, 15 for light to moderate work or exercise, 16.5 for moderate to heavy work or exercise, and 18 for heavy work or exercise.

If you have any specific concerns, we suggest that you seek guidance from a registered, certified, or licensed nutritionist.

Tastes and Smells

Researchers have found that our senses of smell and taste—both of which are often related to food—can also have a significant impact on our dopamine and norepinephrine levels. The *olfactory bulb* (the part of the brain that processes aromas) is closely linked with the limbic system (the part of the brain that processes emotions) and is known to contain almost all the neurotransmitters that are found elsewhere in the brain. Certain aromas can produce changes in brain wave activity as well as the release of neurochemicals. Lemon, basil, peppermint, bitter flavors, and tart foods, for example, make the brain release norepinephrine, which is why lemon scent is often used in aromatherapy to treat loss of energy, mental and physical fatigue, and the inability to concentrate. Hot, spicy foods can have a similar effect, but because they can make you sweat, your body's reaction is to cool itself down by releasing serotonin, which neutralizes the dopamine effect. Recent research indicates that mice who are exposed to rosemary have improved locomotor activity than those who aren't. And several studies have shown that lavender increases penile blood flow and sexual arousal.

Certain odors and scents may actually induce weight loss, according to the neurologist Alan Hirsch, director of the Smell and Taste Treatment and Research Foundation. Since 90 percent of taste is smell, Hirsch decided to investigate whether smelling pleasant food aromas would reduce people's appetite and cravings. He had a number of dieters smell peppermint, green apples, and banana before, during, and after meals and compared their weight loss results. Those who did the most sniffing lost the most weight—and they kept it off too.

Your New Diet and Your Digestion

Changing your diet abruptly will cause some significant changes in the way you digest your food. Most of these changes will be for the positive, helping your stomach and intestines function better and more efficiently.

Sometimes, though, substantially increasing dietary protein and fats (even healthy ones) creates an additional demand for pepsin and other protein-digesting enzymes and stomach acid that your body has not been accustomed to making in the quantity needed to handle your new levels of dietary protein. This relative deficiency of enzymes can create problems digesting your food. If you develop any of the following symptoms, you'll know you need a little temporary help.

- gas
- bloating
- stomach discomfort
- heartburn
- changes in stool, such as what looks like oil in the water, a particularly foul odor, or stools that float

Rather than risk these unpleasant symptoms, there's a simple way to avoid any potential problem: For the first two weeks on your new diet, take one or two tablets of a stomach acid stimulant called *betaine hydrochloride* (or betaine HCL) with every meal that includes higher amounts of protein and/or fat than you're used to. Start weaning yourself off the betaine gradually during the third and fourth weeks of the diet. If you're taking betaine HCL and you develop any of the above symptoms, stop taking it immediately.

Low levels of warming neurotransmitters are sometimes the result of not being able to protect yourself from oxidative stress. The best way of fending off oxidative stress and protecting your warming NT levels is to take antioxidants. These include vitamins C and E, green tea extract (see L-theanine, below), the amino acid acetylcarnitine, and omega-3 fatty acids.

Dietary Supplements

As we discussed above, restructuring your diet is one of the most effective ways of raising your warming neurotransmitter levels. Sometimes, though, you can't do the job by eating normally. In this case you may need to take some nutritional supplements, such as herbs, vitamins, and amino acids. All of these are available over the counter in health food stores and drugstores. While most are safe, we'll point out the ones that you should discuss with your physician before taking.

Herbs

There are two major herbs that boost norepinephrine and/or dopamine levels: ginseng and ginkgo. Both are available at health food and drug-stores everywhere and each acts on a different neurotransmitter. Ginseng works on norepinephrine, so if your symptoms are more physical (lack of energy, fatigue, light-headedness, low blood pressure, weight gain or loss, exercise avoidance, feelings of heat or cold), take that. But if your symptoms are predominately mental and/or emotional (things like difficulties dealing with authority, inability to take pleasure in life, difficulty dealing with frustration) take ginkgo, which has a direct impact on dopamine. If you have physical and mental/emotional symptoms, take both together. Although herbs are generally available over the counter, be sure to check with your doctor (or other health care professional familiar with using herbs as medicine) before taking them. There may be significant negative interactions between certain herbs and other medications you may be taking. Taken under the supervision of a medical professional, these herbs can be extremely effective. Used inappropriately, they can be harmful.

Ginseng.   Medical researchers are paying a lot of attention to ginseng's pharmacological properties and speculate that this herb reduces symptoms of mental exhaustion by increasing dopamine and other heat-producing neurotransmitters in the brain. Increasing heat also raises the body's temperature and burns calories. Ginseng (which is directly translated as "man's essence") has been used for thousands of years as a rejuvenating tonic. In traditional Chinese medicine, ginseng is considered a warming herb. Because it has a vasodilator effect, it is often used to enhance stamina, reduce fatigue, and stimulate the brain, heart, and blood vessels, as well as to treat impotence and erectile dysfunction (both of which are generally blood flow problems). In our practices, we most often recommend it to patients suffering from fatigue or sexual problems. Although its precise mechanism is unclear, some of ginseng's structures and components are similar to those in the heart drug digitalis. Some researchers have suggested that it works by increasing blood flow to various organs, including the brain, heart, and penis. Others have shown that ginseng increases nitric oxide, which produces an effect similar to that of the drug Viagra. For the latter reason we frequently recommend it to counter the sexual side effects of the serotonin-increasing drugs. In animal studies, ginseng extract has been shown to increase immune system function and reduce the length of illnesses. It comes in tablets, capsules, and an alcohol-based tincture. Dosage: 5 mg per pound of body weight (if you weigh 120 pounds you'd take 600 mg per day).

Ginkgo biloba. Ginkgo biloba also raises dopamine and norepinephrine levels indirectly. Scientists have examined the brains of numerous animals (including humans) and have found that the active ingredient in ginkgo biloba works by blocking an enzyme called monoamine oxidase (MAO). MAO's job is to break down dopamine and norepinephrine and get it out of your system. So inhibiting it has the net effect of increasing dopamine levels in the brain. (We'll consider MAO inhibitors in the section on prescription drugs below.) Ginkgo is commonly advertised as a memory-boosting supplement. This is true to a certain extent. By increasing dopamine and blood flow in the area of the brain that governs affective memory, ginkgo makes events seem more worthy of being remembered. In addition, a recent German study found that long-term ginkgo use reduces cardiovascular risks, including those associated with coronary heart disease, hypertension, hypercholesterolemia, and diabetes. Dosage: 60–240 mg per day.

As mentioned earlier, herbs—even though they're available without a prescription—should be taken under the direction of your doctor. If you have high blood pressure or are taking blood thinners or any other MAO inhibitor, *do not* take ginseng or ginkgo without getting an okay from your doctor. Even if you don't have any of those risk factors, both herbs can induce mania if taken in excess.

If You Are Warming Deficient with Diminished Sex Drive or Erectile Dysfunction

Because sexual problems can have a devastating effect on one's psyche and mood, pay close attention to the perspective section of this chapter. It's important that you forgive yourself; worrying and blaming yourself will only make the problem worse. Diet and exercise will also be especially important because they will boost your warming NT levels and your blood flow, both of which may improve your sexual response. You should also:

- Ask your doctor whether any of the prescription medications you're taking could be causing your problems. Blood pressure drugs and many common serotonin-enhancing antidepressants frequently have sexual side effects. Also have him or her check for any vascular problems, including diabetes, which may interrupt blood flow to the sexual organs.
- Take 1,000–3,000 mg per day of vitamin C and 5 mg per day per pound of body weight of ginseng (if you weigh 120 pounds you'll take 600 mg per day).

If reviewing your medications, checking out vascular problems, and taking vitamin C and ginseng don't resolve the issue, ask your doctor about testosterone replacement.

Vitamins

- *Ascorbic acid* (vitamin C) is an essential vitamin. High levels are found in the pituitary and adrenal glands, white blood cells, and the brain. It is a co-factor in the enzyme *tyrosine hydroxylase,* which plays a critical role in synthesizing tyrosine into dopamine and norepinephrine. It is perhaps best known for its antioxidant properties but also has proven effects on iron absorption, immunity, and brain function. It may also reduce the risk of stroke. Increasing vitamin C intake increases dopamine production and has been shown to increase sexual behavior—both frequency and desire. Other studies have found that adults treated with 3 grams (3,000 mg) of vitamin C per day had decreased depression scores and increased libido.
- *Vitamin E* acts as an antioxidant and may stimulate blood flow. Be careful with both vitamins C and E, because in large quantities they may exacerbate bleeding problems, especially if you're on blood-thinning medication.

Amino Acids

Amino acids are the basic building blocks of just about everything in the body. They're involved in making cells, repairing tissue, and helping the body fight infection. They build proteins and carry oxygen through the body. They're also a common nutritional supplement that you can get at a health food or drugstore near you. They come in two types. The *nonessential* variety are the ones your body can manufacture from chemicals already in your system. *Essential* amino acids can't be manufactured internally and have to be brought into the body via food or supplements. Four amino acids have a significant impact on warming neurotransmitters: tyrosine, L-theanine, S-adenosylmethionine (SAM-e), and acetylcarnitine (also called acetyl-L-carnitine). Each of these amino acids acts primarily on a different neurotransmitter: tyrosine and L-theanine on dopamine, SAM-e on norepinephrine, and acetylcarnitine on acetylcholine. If your symptoms are primarily emotional (difficulties dealing with authority, inability to take pleasure in life, frustration, feelings of apathy, lack of interest in sex), you'll want to take tyrosine. If your symptoms are primarily physical (lack of energy, fatigue, light-headedness, low blood pressure, weight gain or loss, always feeling cold), take SAM-e. If your symptoms are primarily mental (memory issues, trouble concentrating, dementia), go with acetylcarnitine. And if you have some combination of any or all of these symptoms, you may need to take more than one amino acid.

L-tyrosine.   An essential amino acid that is the fundamental precursor of both dopamine and norepinephrine. Recent research has shown that it increases the release of dopamine by brain cells. It's found in many foods, particularly those high in protein (such as almonds, avocados, bananas, dairy products, lima beans, pumpkin seeds, and sesame seeds), but even a high-protein diet provides only 100–200 mg per day, which isn't nearly enough. Dosage: 500–1,000 mg as a caffeine alternative to combat fatigue. Tyrosine is very safe.

L-theanine.   Frequently found in green tea. It's marketed in Japan as a nutritional supplement for mood regulation. It releases dopamine in the brain, especially in areas that control mood and memory. A recent Dutch study demonstrated that heavy green tea drinkers had a 68 percent lower risk of heart attack death and a 73 percent lower risk of stroke than non–tea drinkers. In addition, green tea contains a substance called *catechins*, which are powerful antioxidants that block fats in the bloodstream.

S-adenosylmethionine (SAM-e).   A naturally occurring amino acid that is found in every tissue in the body and serves a central role in a number of enzymatic processes. It stimulates dopamine production and blocks the metabolism of norepinephrine (meaning that norepinephrine remains in your system longer). Although sold in the United States only as a dietary supplement, in Europe it's frequently used to treat depression. One recent double-blind study found that 70 percent of those taking SAM-e had significant improvement in mood. In addition, the effects were seen sooner and many of the side effects associated with other antidepressants were avoided. Dosage: For depression, 400–1,600 mg per day. For more minor conditions such as asthma, swelling, hives, and fatigue, 200 mg twice a day on an empty stomach. Caution: Although SAM-e is very safe, it depletes the body's reserves of folic acid and vitamin B-12. So if you're taking SAM-e, be sure to also take 800 mg per day of folic acid and 1,200 mg of B-12 to avoid developing a B-vitamin deficiency.

Acetylcarnitine.   An amino acid that is structurally similar to acetylcholine. It improves cell function by transporting fatty acids into the brain cells, where they're used for energy. It also stimulates the brain's glutamate receptors by increasing blood flow in the brain. People who have taken acetylcarnitine report seeing results—feelings sharper, having more focus, being more alert—often within hours. There are also indications that because acetylcarnitine is used to create acetylcholine, it has certain restorative properties; acetylcholine levels naturally decline as we age. Acetylcarnitine has been successfully used in several double-blind studies to improve symptoms of depression in the elderly and also appears to delay the progression of Alzheimer's disease and has been linked to an increase in cognitive performance in those who already have the disease. A recent study demonstrated that combining acetylcarnitine with the warming antioxidant *alpha-lipoic acid* improved cognition in healthy adults.

If You Are Warming Deficient with Memory Problems

Events make the transition from short-term memory to long-term memory by repetition. Here are a number of things you can do to boost your memory.

- Do things differently. Take a different route to work; vary your routine.
- Keep your mind active. Read anything and everything—especially on subjects you don't know much about. Experiment with new tastes, textures, sights, and sounds that you're not familiar with.
- Turn off the television. Use the time to learn something about a subject that interests you, teach yourself a new language, or spend time in your garden.
- Take some risks. Learn to do something you aren't good at or take a class and force yourself to learn something you think would be a challenge. It doesn't matter what—anything from Thai cooking to mastering the intricacies of neurotransmitter activity in your brain. The point is to learn something new.
- Practice. Whenever you meet someone new, ask his name and then try to use it a few times in your conversation.
- Eat right. Follow the program in this book.
- Exercise. It increases blood flow in your brain and increases the production of dopamine and acetylcholine, both of which play an important role in memory.
- If altering your diet and exercise routine haven't yielded any noticeable result in your memory, try taking 60–240 mg/day of ginkgo (but only if you're not taking any blood-thinning medication) and acetyl-carnitine, which has been shown to increase memory. Before taking either of these compounds, check with your doctor to make sure there won't be any negative reactions.
- If after trying all of the above steps, you're still having memory issues it's time to see your doctor.

Exercise and Activity

Vigorous exercise will increase your dopamine and norepinephrine levels almost immediately, making you feel better and giving you more energy. There are other benefits too. As already noted, the more dopamine and norepinephrine in your system, the more active your natural killer cells will be. Numerous studies have shown that exercising will enhance your immune system and fight off illness and disease, improve your mood, help you lose weight, extend your life span, and even make you smarter.

What's really fascinating is the way this whole process works. Every cell in your body is producing proteins all the time, a certain percentage of which (as with any manufacturing process) are defective in some way. Properly balanced, dopamine and norepinephrine spark the production of specialized proteins called *immunophyllins* or *heat shock proteins,* whose job it is to clean out the defective proteins that clog up your cells and keep them from functioning at their highest level. Some of the cells that get most clogged are the ones responsible for the neurochemistry that stimulates you to exercise. Unfortunately, immunophyllins are very short-lived, which means that you need to produce more of them (by exercising) every few days.

And so, in a kind of vicious cycle, not exercising means you don't produce the heat shock proteins you need to clean out the cells that would send your brain the message that you need to exercise in the first place and give you the willpower to put on your sweats and take those first steps. Exercise also stimulates the production of insulin, which regulates your metabolism (or how active your cells are). The less exercise you do, the less active your cells are, the less energetic you feel, and the less you feel like exercising. Eventually this dynamic can lead to depression and obesity.

Exercise, whether it's running, swimming, skiing, biking, or even just taking a brisk walk, has a clear and almost immediate effect on dopamine. It really doesn't matter what you do, just as long as you do it at least three or four times a week. More often is even better. Your goal should be to raise your heart rate to 80 percent of your predicted maximum and keep it there for twenty to thirty minutes.

Start by choosing a kind of exercise you think you'll enjoy. Do this exercise every day for the duration of this plan. Whether it's Pilates, aerobics, jogging, karate, or dance doesn't matter. What does matter is that you pick something that you'll truly be able to do regularly and that you carefully follow the steps below. You will reap the benefits of exercise by doing something that causes you to sweat each day, even if you are only active for five or ten minutes. It's really about sweating.

While the exercise recommendations in this program may sound painfully simple, exercising in this way will enable you to gradually increase your warming neurotransmitters and your ability to exercise without making your imbalance worse or triggering excess immune system activity. We urge you to be patient and to stick with the program as outlined for the full twenty-eight days. Some of our patients feel so much better after a week on this program that they jump ahead and try to exercise for thirty to forty minutes beyond the point of perspiration. Doing so pushes them beyond their tolerance and often leads to flulike symptoms and exhaustion that can last for three or four days. If you miss more than two consecutive days of exercise, think about starting this part of the plan over from scratch. Rebuilding your tolerance for heat production is best achieved in a gradual and methodical manner. Missing three or four days and picking up where you left off might threaten your program and result in a demoralizing setback.

Sleep

Warming neurotransmitters are what keep your brain active, awake, and capable of concentration and vigilance. Without sufficient warming activity the brain slows down, which allows cooling NTs to dominate. As a warming-deficient person, that is what happened to you. Your brain is struggling to remain alert and unless you consciously take action, you'll fall asleep. Once that happens, you're probably difficult to arouse. You may need ten to twelve hours of sleep a night and still wake up tired, or you may find yourself wanting a nap in the middle of the day.

This kind of excessive sleepiness or tiredness is very common in our fast-paced society. It can also be one of the major symptoms of depression. However, this is very different from some more serious sleep-related conditions such as narcolepsy, which is caused by an actual brain abnormality. Narcoleptics are often excessively tired during the day and sometimes suffer from attacks of "microsleep," where they suddenly and unexpectedly fall asleep for a few minutes wherever they are.

If You Are Warming Deficient with Extreme Fatigue

If you're exhausted, you may be too tired to bother with perspective and worldview and exercise. You may not even be particularly hungry, but chances are you're going to eat at some point. When you do, make an effort to stay on the diet we outlined here and add the following:

- 500–1,000 mg per day of tyrosine
- 5 mg per day per pound of body weight of ginseng (if you weigh 120 pounds, you'll take 600 mg per day)
- 1,000–3,000 mg per day of vitamin C

Try to incorporate as many of the warming-enhancing lifestyle changes suggested in this chapter as possible. When you're feeling well enough to exercise, get yourself on a regular program such as the one outlined here. Be *very* careful not to overdo it, or you'll end up feeling worse than you do now. If you follow these steps and still aren't feeling less fatigued within a week, we recommend that you ask your doctor to order a complete blood chemistry workup, including thyroid and testosterone (even if you're a woman). Ask whether he or she thinks Provigil would be appropriate for you.

Putting It All Together: The 28-Day Warming Program

WEEK ONE

The theme for this week is to change your internal dialogues. Replace all those I can'ts with I cans or at least I'll trys. When you become aware of negative thoughts creeping into your brain, don't panic. Be aware of them and slowly try to replace them with something more positive. And don't let previous mistakes undermine your trust in yourself. Your intuition isn't as bad as you may think.

Although a lot of people might think that there's no such thing as too much sleep, the opposite is true. More than eight hours a night can actually be harmful and may increase your risk of heart attack. This week, any time you feel tired, do something that increases your activity level: run, stretch, jump up and down, or go for a quick walk. This will increase warming NT production and raise your energy levels.

This week we'll also introduce three vitamin, herb, and amino acid combinations that will be the foundation of your nutritional supplement program for the rest of the 28-day program. These are:

- The Advanced Brain Chemistry (ABC) Antioxidant Mixture, which consists of
  - 400 IU vitamin E
  - 500 mg slow-release vitamin C

- The Advanced Brain Chemistry (ABC) Warming Herb Mixture, which consists of
  - 60 mg of ginkgo
  - 40 mg of ginseng
  - 100 mg of green tea extract
- The Advanced Brain Chemistry (ABC) Warming Amino Mixture, which consists of
  - 250 mg of tyrosine
  - 250 mg of acetylcarnitine (sometimes called AL-carnitine)

Day 1

Perspective

Today's mission statement: I am strong, confident, and capable, and I can do whatever I set my mind to.

Lifestyle

Create a new morning routine. Your brain and body get bored doing the same thing every day. Anything you can do to shake things up a little will give you a jolt of warming neurotransmitters.

Diet and Supplements

Throughout the day—with and between meals—drink one half ounce of liquid per pound of body weight (if you weigh 130 pounds, that's 65 ounces). But no matter how much you weigh, make sure you get a minimum of 64 ounces. Water, green tea, cinnamon-spiced tea, and oolong tea are excellent choices; caffeinated drinks, alcohol, and fruit juices don't count.

BREAKFAST

    Vegetable omelet:

           3 whole eggs and 3 egg whites

           1 T. onion, diced

           1 T. green pepper, diced

           2 oz. low-fat cheddar cheese, crumbled

    1 orange

SNACK

    1 low-carb (less than 5 grams of sugar) protein bar

LUNCH

Turkey salad:

5 oz. sliced turkey breast

3 T. diced celery

2 T. diced carrots

1½ T. reduced-fat mayonnaise

1 large apple

SNACK

1 cup of low-calorie cocoa made with low-fat or skim milk

DINNER

5 oz. steak

1 c. brown rice

2 c. broccoli

3 c. tossed salad

1 T. low-fat dressing

SUPPLEMENTS

- 1 ABC Antioxidant Mixture, twice a day with food
- 1 ABC Warming Herb Mixture, twice a day (Take one hour before eating or two hours after.)
- 2 ABC Warming Amino Mixture, twice a day

Exercise

Exercise to the point of sweating, then stop. Your workout is over for the day.

Sleep

Sleep no longer than seven and a half or eight hours. If you need to, get an alarm clock with the most annoying buzzer you can find or tune the radio to a music station you really hate. Put it far enough away from your bed that you'll have to get up to turn it off.

Day 2

Perspective

I can—and I do—make a difference.

Reducing Your Hunger Pangs by Going Nuts

For the first week or so after you start reducing your caloric intake, you may get hit with some powerful feelings of hunger. We've found that you can overcome food cravings through using a two-pronged approach:

1. Visualize your ideal self. How are you going to look physically when you've reached your ideal size? Associate this visualization with the rewards it will bring you. Visualize your improved self doing something pleasurable with someone you find attractive and fit.
2. Have a handful of nuts—almonds, pecans, macadamia nuts, and/or walnuts. Nuts are full of beneficial omega-3 fatty acids, and a handful (be reasonable) can suppress your appetite for 2½ hours. A number of studies have shown that nuts are great for other reasons too.
   - People who ate twenty-five almonds a day for a month reduced their LDL (bad) cholesterol by 4 percent and raised their HDL (good) cholesterol by 5 percent.
   - Vegetarians who eat 2 ounces of nuts four to five times a week had half the heart attack risk of those who didn't eat nuts at all.
   - A 1-ounce serving of nuts five or more times a week led to a 27 percent reduction in risk for type 2 diabetes. Eating peanut butter instead of nuts reduced the risk by almost 20 percent.

Lifestyle

Take a cool shower and dry off vigorously. Dopamine and norepinephrine heat the body. Exposure to cold drops your body temperature a little bit, which causes your brain to release enough dopamine to raise it back up again.

Diet and Supplements

Throughout the day—with and between meals—drink one half ounce of liquid per pound of body weight (if you weigh 130 pounds, that's 65 ounces). But no matter how much you weigh, make sure you get a

minimum of 64 ounces. Water, green tea, cinnamon-spiced tea, and oolong tea are excellent choices; caffeinated drinks, alcohol, and fruit juices don't count.

BREAKFAST

> 1¼ c. low-fat cottage cheese
>
> 2 medium apples, diced
>
> 1½ T. diced cashews

SNACK

> 2 celery stalks stuffed with low-fat cream cheese or peanut butter

LUNCH

> Caesar salad:
>> 4.5 oz. chicken breast
>>
>> 1 t. grated parmesan cheese
>>
>> 4 c. red leaf lettuce
>>
>> 1½ T. Caesar dressing, bottled
>
> 12 grapes

SNACK

> 1 low-carb (less than 5 grams of sugar) protein bar

DINNER

> 5 oz. lean pork tenderloin
>
> 2 T. barbecue sauce
>
> 1½ c. coleslaw
>
> 1 c. green beans
>
> ½ c. peaches

SUPPLEMENTS

- 1 ABC Antioxidant Mixture, twice a day with food
- 1 ABC Warming Herb Mixture, twice a day (Take one hour before eating or two hours after.)
- 2 ABC Warming Amino Mixture, twice a day

Exercise

Exercise until you notice that you're sweating, then go one more minute. That's it.

Sleep

Sleep no more than seven and a half or eight hours. In the morning, take a cool shower and dry off vigorously to rinse the cobwebs out of your eyes and get your blood flowing.

Day 3

Perspective

If I do not create myself, someone else will.

Lifestyle

Listen to some rap music or music with a fast beat—especially if you don't like it. This kind of music stimulates electrical impulses in our inner ears, which in turn stimulates the brain to produce the kind of high-frequency brain waves that trigger dopamine and norepinephrine release. The rhythm may make you rock your head, tap your feet, and eventually get up and dance. All of these activities increase norepinephrine and dopamine levels.

Diet and Supplements

Throughout the day—with and between meals—drink one half ounce of liquid per pound of body weight (if you weigh 130 pounds, that's 65 ounces). But no matter how much you weigh, make sure you get a minimum of 64 ounces. Water, green tea, cinnamon-spiced tea, and oolong tea are excellent choices; caffeinated drinks, alcohol, and fruit juices don't count.

BREAKFAST

    1 c. slow-cooked oatmeal

    ½ c. low-fat milk

    1½ T. diced almonds

    1 t. honey

    1 small apple

SNACK

    ½ c. fresh fruit and 1 oz. cheddar cheese

LUNCH

Tuna salad:

    5 oz. tuna

    ½ celery stalk, diced

    1 T. onion, diced

    3 T. low-fat mayonnaise

1 small pickle

1 medium orange

SNACK

2 T. peanut butter on celery sticks

DINNER

4.5 oz. salmon

Grilled vegetables (grilled in nonstick skillet):

    4 onion slices

    1 red pepper

    1 zucchini

    1 T. dressing for marinade

2 c. tossed salad

SUPPLEMENTS

- 1 ABC Antioxidant Mixture, twice a day with food
- 1 ABC Warming Herb Mixture, twice a day (Take one hour before eating or two hours after.)
- 2 ABC Warming Amino Mixture, twice a day

Exercise

Exercise until you notice that you're sweating, then go two more minutes.

Sleep

Sleep no more than seven and a half or eight hours. In the morning, do a few minutes of gentle stretching before you get out of bed to stimulate warming neurotransmitter production.

Day 4

Perspective

If not now, when? If I am not for myself, who will be?

Lifestyle

Concentrate hard today. Focusing—whether it's on the *New York Times* crossword puzzle, having a fascinating conversation, or doing an elaborate spreadsheet—raises norepinephrine levels and warms the brain.

Diet and Supplements

Throughout the day—with and between meals—drink one half ounce of liquid per pound of body weight (if you weigh 130 pounds, that's 65 ounces). But no matter how much you weigh, make sure you get a minimum of 64 ounces. Water, green tea, cinnamon-spiced tea, and oolong tea are excellent choices; caffeinated drinks, alcohol, and fruit juices don't count.

BREAKFAST

Scrambled cheese eggs:

3 whole eggs and 3 egg whites

1 oz. cheddar cheese

1 grapefruit

SNACK

1 cup of low-calorie cocoa made with low-fat or skim milk

LUNCH

6 oz. lean roast beef

2 slices tomato

2 large lettuce leaves

1½ T. low-fat mayonnaise

1 small tangerine

SNACK

6 oz. nonfat yogurt with fruit

DINNER

Sauté with soy sauce to taste:

  ¾ c. low-fat tofu

  1 c. red peppers

  1 c. broccoli

  1 T. olive oil

1 c. brown rice

2 c. tossed salad

1 T. low-fat salad dressing

SUPPLEMENTS

- 1 ABC Antioxidant Mixture, twice a day with food
- 1 ABC Warming Herb Mixture, twice a day (Take one hour before eating or two hours after.)
- 2 ABC Warming Amino Mixture, twice a day

Exercise

Exercise until you notice that you're sweating, and then go three more minutes.

Sleep

Sleep no more than seven and a half or eight hours. Get some fresh air first thing in the morning. A short walk is great; so is taking a few deep breaths of cold air in your own backyard.

Day 5

Perspective

I know I can handle anything, no matter how hard, as long as I take it slowly.

Lifestyle

Do something physical around the house. Put up those bookshelves you've been thinking about. Paint the bathroom, trim the trees, clean out the garage, or mow the lawn with a manual mower.

Diet and Supplements

Throughout the day—with and between meals—drink one half ounce of liquid per pound of body weight (if you weigh 130 pounds, that's 65 ounces). But no matter how much you weigh, make sure you get a

minimum of 64 ounces. Water, green tea, cinnamon-spiced tea, and oolong tea are excellent choices; caffeinated drinks, alcohol, and fruit juices don't count.

Breakfast

8 oz. low-fat yogurt without fruit

3 pieces Canadian bacon

1 T. almonds

Snack

½ c. roasted soy nuts

Lunch

5 oz. grilled chicken breast

2 slices tomato

2 large lettuce leaves

1 T. ketchup

Snack

1 low-carb (less than 5 grams sugar) protein bar

Dinner

5 oz. lean ground beef

1 c. chopped lettuce

4 T. diced tomato

½ small diced carrot

2 T. low-fat dressing

Supplements

- 1 ABC Antioxidant Mixture, twice a day with food
- 1 ABC Warming Herb Mixture, twice a day (Take one hour before eating or two hours after.)
- 2 ABC Warming Amino Mixture, twice a day

Exercise

Exercise until you notice that you're sweating, then go four more minutes.

Sleep

Sleep no more than seven and a half to eight hours. Before sleeping, instead of reading the newspaper, which is often filled with really depressing articles, read something you find inspiring and uplifting.

Day 6

Perspective

Today I will be optimistic. I will not allow negative thoughts to intrude.

Lifestyle

Pay attention to your posture and sit up straight all day long. That may sound silly, but slouching can press on veins that take blood to the brain, causing fuzzy thinking and forgetfulness—two classic warming deficit symptoms.

Diet and Supplements

Throughout the day—with and between meals—drink one half ounce of liquid per pound of body weight (if you weigh 130 pounds, that's 65 ounces). But no matter how much you weigh, make sure you get a minimum of 64 ounces. Water, green tea, cinnamon-spiced tea, and oolong tea are excellent choices; caffeinated drinks, alcohol, and fruit juices don't count.

BREAKFAST

    4 oz. lean ham

    1 slice skim mozzarella

    1 small apple

SNACK

    8 oz. protein shake (make 16 oz. in blender and drink 8 oz. now)

        whey protein powder, vanilla flavor (8 grams of protein)

        1 medium banana

        1 c. strawberries

        2 T. almonds

LUNCH

    5 slices low-fat cheese

    3 slices tomato

1 small carrot

1 small pickle

SNACK

Remaining 8 oz. of protein shake

DINNER

4.5 oz. grilled halibut

⅔ c. brown rice

10 asparagus spears

2 c. tossed salad

1½ T. low-fat dressing

½ c. peaches

SUPPLEMENTS

- 1 ABC Antioxidant Mixture, twice a day with food
- 1 ABC Warming Herb Mixture, twice a day (Take one hour before eating or two hours after.)
- 2 ABC Warming Amino Mixture, twice a day

Exercise

Exercise until you notice that you're sweating, then go five more minutes.

Sleep

Sleep no more than seven and a half to eight hours. In the morning, don't skip breakfast. It's an important start to the day.

Day 7

Perspective

I alone am the one who can make me happy.

Lifestyle

Eat something extremely tart today. Lemon, basil, peppermint, bitter flavors, and tart foods release dopamine and norepinephrine in the brain. These scents in particular have been shown to increase energy, blood flow, and concentration.

Diet and Supplements

Throughout the day—with and between meals—drink one half ounce of liquid per pound of body weight (if you weigh 130 pounds, that's 65 ounces). But no matter how much you weigh, make sure you get a minimum of 64 ounces. Water, green tea, cinnamon-spiced tea, and oolong tea are excellent choices; caffeinated drinks, alcohol, and fruit juices don't count.

BREAKFAST

>2 slices low-fat cheese
>
>5 oz. sliced turkey
>
>½ orange

SNACK

>3 oz. water-pack tuna
>
>3 carrot sticks
>
>1 c. chopped iceberg lettuce

LUNCH

>4.5 oz. grilled chicken breast
>
>½ c. chopped broccoli
>
>1 c. tossed salad
>
>3 T. regular dressing
>
>1 small apple

SNACK

>6 oz. fat-free banana yogurt

DINNER

>6 oz. grilled veal chops
>
>1 c. red peppers
>
>1 c. mushrooms
>
>3 c. spinach
>
>2 T. low-fat dressing
>
>½ c. applesauce

SUPPLEMENTS

- 1 ABC Antioxidant Mixture, twice a day with food
- 1 ABC Warming Herb Mixture, twice a day (Take one hour before eating or two hours after.)
- 2 ABC Warming Amino Mixture, twice a day

Exercise

Exercise until you notice that you're sweating, then go six more minutes.

Sleep

Sleep no more than seven and a half to eight hours. After almost a week, it's safe to change the station on your clock radio. Wake up to some upbeat music, *not* news.

WEEK TWO

This week's theme is to get to know more positive people and surround yourself with people who will support your commitment to your goals. Malcontents are always looking for someone to drag themselves down with. Hang out with some good friends. People with social networks and confidants they can share their feelings and concerns with are healthier, get sick less often, recover more quickly, and live longer.

This week we'll make some small changes to your supplement regime, and you'll continue adding one minute per day to your exercise routine.

If you're still tired or sleepy or can't wake up without feeling that you need another hour in bed, get more light. Our warming NTs are naturally overwhelmed in the evening by cooling activity. Sunset, even when skies are cloudy, affects an area of the brain called the *pineal gland,* which releases melatonin, a cooling antioxidant. Melatonin increases the activity of substance S and other sleep-inducing chemicals and eventually puts you to sleep. Warming NT-deficient people have a defect in this system and often "leak" melatonin from the pineal gland during the day. Sunlight or artificial, full-spectrum Ott lighting can suppress the release of melatonin and postpone the onset of sleep. Unless you already spend a lot of time outdoors, consider installing full-spectrum lighting in your home or office.

Day 8

Perspective

Today's mission statement is: I accept only acceptable behavior toward me and I have the right to tell people how to treat me well.

Lifestyle

Buy a sex toy or rent an x-rated movie and enjoy them with a friend or alone. If you're not in a relationship, simply fantasizing about sex will increase your dopamine levels.

Diet and Supplements

Throughout the day—with and between meals—drink one half ounce of liquid per pound of body weight (if you weigh 130 pounds, that's 65 ounces). But no matter how much you weigh, make sure you get a minimum of 64 ounces. Water, green tea, cinnamon-spiced tea, and oolong tea are excellent choices; caffeinated drinks, alcohol, and fruit juices don't count.

BREAKFAST

2 poached eggs

1 c. cottage cheese

1 peach

SNACK

1 apple

LUNCH

2 c. stir-fry vegetables (carrots, zucchini, broccoli)

1 c. brown rice

1 peach or plum

SNACK

1 T. peanut butter on apple slices

DINNER

1 c. low-fat turkey chili

1 c. steamed green beans

1 bottle nonalcoholic beer

SUPPLEMENTS

- 2 ABC Antioxidant Mixture, twice a day with food
- 2 ABC Warming Herb Mixture, twice a day (Take one hour before eating or two hours after.)
- 2 ABC Warming Amino Mixture, three times a day

Exercise

Exercise until you notice that you're sweating, then go seven more minutes.

Sleep

Sleep no more than seven and a half to eight hours. Throw open the shades first thing in the morning and let the sun in.

Day 9

Perspective

I have the strength to say what needs to be said and to listen to others, even when I don't agree with them.

Lifestyle

Take some action. You can't make a physical move of any kind without a spurt of dopamine. Even the process of simply *imagining* that you're going to get up stimulates just enough dopamine and norepinephrine to give you the energy to get off the couch. Actually getting up produces even more. Even tightly gripping the armrest of your chair for thirty seconds will have an effect.

Diet and Supplements

Throughout the day—with and between meals—drink one half ounce of liquid per pound of body weight (if you weigh 130 pounds, that's 65 ounces). But no matter how much you weigh, make sure you get a minimum of 64 ounces. Water, green tea, cinnamon-spiced tea, and oolong tea are excellent choices; caffeinated drinks, alcohol, and fruit juices don't count.

BREAKFAST

3 slices low-fat deli turkey, pan seared

2 oz. low-fat cheddar cheese

2 grapefruit halves

SNACK

   ½ c. roasted pumpkin seeds

LUNCH

   5 oz. chicken breast

   1 c. steamed broccoli

   small green salad with carrots and tomato slices

SNACK

   Berry smoothie:

   ½ scoop whey protein powder

   ½ c. blueberries or mixed berries

   4 oz. orange juice

   4 oz. nonfat milk

DINNER

   6 oz. smoked chicken

   2 c. cooked lentils

   8–10 brussels sprouts

SUPPLEMENTS

   * 2 ABC Antioxidant Mixture, twice a day with food
   * 2 ABC Warming Herb Mixture, twice a day (Take one hour before eating or two hours after.)
   * 2 ABC Warming Amino Mixture, three times a day

Exercise

Exercise until you notice that you're sweating, then go eight more minutes.

Sleep

Keep implementing the strategies from week 1 to limit your sleep to seven and a half to eight hours.

Day 10

Perspective

I have the courage to ask for help and emotional support when I need it.

Lifestyle

Watch something fast, such as auto races, football, or hockey. In another primitive reaction, our brain perceives things that move as threats and responds by kicking in our sympathetic nervous system, which increases blood pressure, pulse, and raises our levels of awareness—all of which require dopamine and norepinephrine.

Diet and Supplements

Throughout the day—with and between meals—drink one half ounce of liquid per pound of body weight (if you weigh 130 pounds, that's 65 ounces). But no matter how much you weigh, make sure you get a minimum of 64 ounces. Water, green tea, cinnamon-spiced tea, and oolong tea are excellent choices; caffeinated drinks, alcohol, and fruit juices don't count.

BREAKFAST
> 1 c. all-bran cereal
>
> 1 c. milk
>
> 1 orange, sliced

SNACK
> Protein shake:
>> whey protein powder, vanilla flavor (8 grams of protein)
>>
>> 1 medium banana
>>
>> 1 c. strawberries
>>
>> 2 T. almonds

LUNCH
> Turkey salad:
>> 5 oz. turkey breast
>>
>> ½ celery stalk, sliced
>>
>> 1 t. onion, diced
>>
>> 1 T. low-fat mayonnaise
>
> 4 oz. grapes

SNACK
> Handful of macadamia nuts

DINNER

> 8 oz. grilled tofu steaks
>
> Romaine lettuce salad with chopped carrots, 1 T. olive oil
>
> 1 c. mushrooms
>
> 4 oz. steamed broccoli

SUPPLEMENTS

- 2 ABC Antioxidant Mixture, twice a day with food
- 2 ABC Warming Herb Mixture, twice a day (Take one hour before eating or two hours after.)
- 2 ABC Warming Amino Mixture, three times a day

Exercise

Exercise until you notice that you're sweating, then go nine more minutes.

Sleep

Keep implementing the strategies from week 1 to limit your sleep to seven and a half to eight hours.

Day 11

Perspective

I will seek to understand rather than to be understood.

Lifestyle

Make a realistic to-do list and force yourself to accomplish as many of the day's goals as you can.

Diet and Supplements

Throughout the day—with and between meals—drink one half ounce of liquid per pound of body weight (if you weigh 130 pounds, that's 65 ounces). But no matter how much you weigh, make sure you get a minimum of 64 ounces. Water, green tea, cinnamon-spiced tea, and oolong tea are excellent choices; caffeinated drinks, alcohol, and fruit juices don't count.

BREAKFAST

    1 c. oatmeal with almonds

    ½ cantaloupe

    2 scrambled eggs

SNACK

    6 oz. nonfat yogurt with fruit

LUNCH

    3 oz. water-pack tuna with 1 T. low-fat mayonnaise

    1 c. sliced tomatoes

    ½ avocado

SNACK

    ¼ c. roasted soy nuts

    ¼ c. golden raisins

DINNER

    6 oz. broiled filet of sole

    1 c. spinach salad with olive oil, garlic, lemon juice

    4 asparagus spears

SUPPLEMENTS

- 2 ABC Antioxidant Mixture, twice a day with food
- 2 ABC Warming Herb Mixture, twice a day (Take one hour before eating or two hours after.)
- 2 ABC Warming Amino Mixture, three times a day

Exercise

Exercise until you notice that you're sweating, then go ten more minutes.

Sleep

Keep implementing the strategies from week 1 to limit your sleep to seven and a half to eight hours.

Day 12

Perspective

I congratulate myself on the steps I'm taking to change and improve my life.

Lifestyle

Do something that makes you nervous or that challenges you. If you hate public speaking, make a presentation to your coworkers. If you're single and shy, ask out someone you've admired. If you're married, tell your spouse a secret you've never told anyone before. Maybe even sign up for a survival course.

Diet and Supplements

Throughout the day—with and between meals—drink one half ounce of liquid per pound of body weight (if you weigh 130 pounds, that's 65 ounces). But no matter how much you weigh, make sure you get a minimum of 64 ounces. Water, green tea, cinnamon-spiced tea, and oolong tea are excellent choices; caffeinated drinks, alcohol, and fruit juices don't count.

BREAKFAST

Herb omelet

1 oz. cheese

3 slices turkey bacon

SNACK

Handful of almonds

LUNCH

4 oz. baked chicken breast

1 c. brown rice

1 c. steamed summer squash

SNACK

1 c. fresh strawberries with nonfat whipped cream

DINNER

  4 oz. steamed salmon

  1 c. pasta salad with olive oil vinaigrette

  1 c. roasted potatoes seasoned with garlic

SUPPLEMENTS

- 2 ABC Antioxidant Mixture, twice a day with food
- 2 ABC Warming Herb Mixture, twice a day (Take one hour before eating or two hours after.)
- 2 ABC Warming Amino Mixture, three times a day

Exercise

Exercise until you notice that you're sweating, then go eleven more minutes.

Sleep

Keep implementing the strategies from week 1 to limit your sleep to seven and a half to eight hours.

Day 13

Perspective

I am in control of my thoughts and I can overcome any adversity.

Lifestyle

Get up half an hour early. You'll be a little more tired than usual, and your brain will try to help you out with a little dose of energizing dopamine and norepinephrine.

Diet and Supplements

Throughout the day—with and between meals—drink one half ounce of liquid per pound of body weight (if you weigh 130 pounds, that's 65 ounces). But no matter how much you weigh, make sure you get a minimum of 64 ounces. Water, green tea, cinnamon-spiced tea, and oolong tea are excellent choices; caffeinated drinks, alcohol, and fruit juices don't count.

BREAKFAST

  3 slices smoked salmon

  1 apple, sliced

SNACK

1 fresh pear

LUNCH

Chicken Caesar salad

6 carrot sticks

½ cantaloupe

SNACK

1 low-carb (less than 5 grams of sugar) protein bar

DINNER

6 oz. grilled lean pork tenderloin

2 c. steamed cauliflower and green beans

1 c. canned peaches, drained, with fruit juice

SUPPLEMENTS

- 2 ABC Antioxidant Mixture, twice a day with food
- 2 ABC Warming Herb Mixture, twice a day (Take one hour before eating or two hours after.)
- 2 ABC Warming Amino Mixture, three times a day

Exercise

Exercise until you notice that you're sweating, then go twelve more minutes.

Sleep

Keep implementing the strategies from week 1 to limit your sleep to seven and a half to eight hours.

Day 14

Perspective

I have the right to have relationships with people who love and support me, and I surround myself with people just like that.

Lifestyle

Sing, shout, or make some noise. Norepinephrine is what keeps us alert and on our toes. Loud noises make the brain release norepinephrine so we can sit up and pay attention.

Diet and Supplements

Throughout the day—with and between meals—drink one half ounce of liquid per pound of body weight (if you weigh 130 pounds, that's 65 ounces). But no matter how much you weigh, make sure you get a minimum of 64 ounces. Water, green tea, cinnamon-spiced tea, and oolong tea are excellent choices; caffeinated drinks, alcohol, and fruit juices don't count.

BREAKFAST

    1 c. high-fiber cereal

    1 c. skim milk

    ½ grapefruit, sweetened to taste with stevia (available at your health food store)

SNACK

    6 oz. sugar-free, fat-free blueberry yogurt

LUNCH

    5 oz. low-fat ham

    low-fat mayonnaise, Dijon mustard, lettuce, tomato

    green salad with 1 T. fat-free dressing

    1 small apple

SNACK

    ½ c. roasted soy nuts

DINNER

    1 serving low-carb pasta

    ½ c. spaghetti sauce w/mushrooms

    2 T. grated cheese

    ¾ c. snap peas

    green salad with 1 T. olive oil and 1 T. lemon juice

    1 c. fresh pineapple slices

SUPPLEMENTS

- 2 ABC Antioxidant Mixture, twice a day with food
- 2 ABC Warming Herb Mixture, twice a day (Take one hour before eating or two hours after.)
- 2 ABC Warming Amino Mixture, three times a day

Exercise

Exercise until you notice that you're sweating, then go thirteen more minutes.

Sleep

Keep implementing the strategies from week 1 to limit your sleep to seven and a half to eight hours.

WEEK THREE

This week's theme is to think things through. When facing a choice—and there's almost always a choice—go over your options carefully. If you need some advice, get it. You don't have to do everything by yourself. Once you've gathered enough information, make your decision and do what needs to be done.

If you've been eating right and exercising regularly for the past few weeks, you'll probably notice that you don't need as much sleep as you used to and that the quality of your sleep is better. However, you still may not be as energetic as you'd like to be. If so, don't be afraid to take a little snooze. An occasional catnap can prove surprisingly refreshing and allow you to burn off some of those excess cooling NTs and restore a better warming-cooling balance. Take quick naps as often as you need to, but don't sleep any longer than fifteen minutes. (Fifteen to twenty minutes after you fall asleep, your brain shifts from stage 1 non-REM sleep to stage 2 non-REM sleep, from which it's a lot harder to awaken.)

Day 15

Perspective

Today's mission statement is: I have the right to consider my options before making a decision.

Lifestyle

Try a food you've never eaten but have heard unpleasant things about. Come on, admit it. You've always wanted to taste limburger cheese, haven't you? And then there's durian, a fruit that smells like rotting flesh. It's incredibly popular in Asia and you can probably buy one at a Chinatown near you. And there's always liver.

Diet and Supplements

Throughout the day—with and between meals—drink one half ounce of liquid per pound of body weight (if you weigh 130 pounds, that's 65 ounces). But no matter how much you weigh, make sure you get a minimum of 64 ounces. Water, green tea, cinnamon-spiced tea, and oolong tea are excellent choices; caffeinated drinks, alcohol, and fruit juices don't count.

BREAKFAST

8 ounces protein shake (make 16 oz. in blender and drink 8 oz. now)
> 1⅓ c. low-fat yogurt
> 1 scoop whey protein powder
> 1 T. almonds

SNACK

Remaining 8 oz. protein shake

LUNCH

1 medium russet potato topped with:
> 2 oz. shredded jack cheese
> ½ c. broccoli
> ½ c. chopped carrots

1 c. pineapple chunks

SNACK

½ c. blueberries

DINNER

2 Boca burger patties (available at most healthfood stores)

2 slices tomato

2 large lettuce leaves

1 T. ketchup

SUPPLEMENTS

- 2 ABC Antioxidant Mixture, twice a day with food
- 2 ABC Warming Herb Mixture, twice a day (Take one hour before eating or two hours after.)

- 3 ABC Warming Amino Mixture, three times a day
- 200 mg SAM-e, twice a day, upon awakening and at midmorning

Exercise

Exercise until you notice that you're sweating, then go fourteen more minutes.

Sleep

Take a short nap if you have to and keep implementing the strategies from weeks 1 and 2 to limit your sleep to a good seven and a half to eight hours.

Day 16

Perspective

Risk is a part of life. I am willing to take risks even when I am afraid.

Lifestyle

Do a virtual workout. In a fascinating recent experiment, researchers at the Cleveland Clinic Foundation found that people can strengthen their muscles just by thinking about it. They had a group of thirty young adults imagine, as realistically as possible, using either their elbow flexor or the muscle of their little finger for five minutes a day, five times a week for twelve weeks. A control group did no imaginary exercise at all. The imaginary exercises increased elbow strength by over 13 percent and baby finger flexing power by 35 percent. Researchers also found more brain-wave activity in the prefrontal cortex after the twelve-week imaginary workout than before it started.

Diet and Supplements

Throughout the day—with and between meals—drink one half ounce of liquid per pound of body weight (if you weigh 130 pounds, that's 65 ounces). But no matter how much you weigh, make sure you get a minimum of 64 ounces. Water, green tea, cinnamon-spiced tea, and oolong tea are excellent choices; caffeinated drinks, alcohol, and fruit juices don't count.

BREAKFAST

   2 scrambled eggs

   3 strips reduced-fat turkey bacon

   ½ grapefruit

   1 c. skim milk

SNACK

   1 oz. cheese

LUNCH

   6 oz. baked cod steak

   1 c. steamed broccoli

   ½ c. fresh fruit cocktail

SNACK

   1 low-carb (less than 5 grams of sugar) protein bar

DINNER

   3–4 oz. grilled pork loin chop

   1 c. steamed rice

   1 c. spinach

   1 c. cooked carrots

   ½ c. canned peaches in fruit juice

SUPPLEMENTS

- 2 ABC Antioxidant Mixture, twice a day with food
- 2 ABC Warming Herb Mixture, twice a day (Take one hour before eating or two hours after.)
- 3 ABC Warming Amino Mixture, three times a day
- 200 mg SAM-e, twice a day, upon awakening and at midmorning

Exercise

Exercise until you notice that you're sweating, then go fifteen more minutes.

Sleep

Take a short nap if you have to, and keep implementing the strategies from weeks 1 and 2 to limit your sleep to a good seven and a half to eight hours.

Day 17

Perspective

I have the right to set limits and the courage to do so.

Lifestyle

Get something off your chest that's really bothered you. Standing up for yourself or for something you feel is wrong will trigger a healthy release of dopamine.

Diet and Supplements

Throughout the day—with and between meals—drink one half ounce of liquid per pound of body weight (if you weigh 130 pounds, that's 65 ounces). But no matter how much you weigh, make sure you get a minimum of 64 ounces. Water, green tea, cinnamon-spiced tea, and oolong tea are excellent choices; caffeinated drinks, alcohol, and fruit juices don't count.

BREAKFAST

2 whole grain low-carb pancakes

½ c. sugar-free fruit compote

1 c. low-fat milk

SNACK

1 flour tortilla (low-carb if possible)

1 oz. low-fat cheddar cheese

1 T. salsa

LUNCH

4 oz. low-fat sliced turkey breast

2 slices jack cheese

tomato slices, lettuce

1 T. low-fat mayonnaise, 1 t. vinegar

1 c. mandarin oranges

SNACK

  1 c. fresh strawberries with nonfat whipped cream

DINNER

  1 barbecued chicken breast

  ½ c. fresh fruit cocktail

  ½ pint cole slaw

SUPPLEMENTS

- 2 ABC Antioxidant Mixture, twice a day with food
- 2 ABC Warming Herb Mixture, twice a day (Take one hour before eating or two hours after.)
- 3 ABC Warming Amino Mixture, three times a day
- 200 mg SAM-e, twice a day, upon awakening and at midmorning

Exercise

Exercise until you notice that you're sweating, then go sixteen more minutes.

Sleep

Take a short nap if you have to and keep implementing the strategies from weeks 1 and 2 to limit your sleep to a good seven and a half to eight hours.

Day 18

Perspective

I will make time to do things I want to do in addition to the things I have to do.

Lifestyle

Rent a scary movie—another great way to give your fight-or-flight system a workout.

Diet and Supplements

Throughout the day—with and between meals—drink one half ounce of liquid per pound of body weight (if you weigh 130 pounds, that's 65 ounces). But no matter how much you weigh, make sure you get a

minimum of 64 ounces. Water, green tea, cinnamon-spiced tea, and oolong tea are excellent choices; caffeinated drinks, alcohol, and fruit juices don't count.

BREAKFAST

2 poached eggs

1 banana

SNACK

Blueberry-strawberry smoothie:
  ¼ c. blueberries
  ¼ c. strawberries
  ½ scoop whey protein powder (8 grams of protein)
  3 oz. orange juice
  3 oz. nonfat milk

LUNCH

1 serving low-carb pasta

½ c. spaghetti sauce with mushrooms

2 T. grated cheese

¾ c. snap peas

green salad with 1 T. olive oil and 1 T. lemon juice

1 c. pineapple slices

SNACK

1 oz. nuts

DINNER

6 oz. steamed filet of orange roughy

1 c. steamed broccoli

½ c. fruit cocktail

SUPPLEMENTS

- 2 ABC Antioxidant Mixture, twice a day with food
- 2 ABC Warming Herb Mixture, twice a day (Take one hour before eating or two hours after.)
- 3 ABC Warming Amino Mixture, three times a day
- 200 mg SAM-e, twice a day, upon awakening and at midmorning

Exercise

Exercise until you notice that you're sweating, then go seventeen more minutes.

Sleep

Take a short nap if you have to, and keep implementing the strategies from weeks 1 and 2 to limit your sleep to a good seven and a half to eight hours.

Day 19

Perspective

I am in control of my own life and I make the choices about how I act at any given moment.

Lifestyle

Get some fresh air first thing in the morning or whenever you're feeling tired, or take a cool shower and dry off vigorously. Your brain responds to your body's drop in temperature by pumping out enough dopamine to restore warmth. In the process you get a little more energy.

Diet and Supplements

Throughout the day—with and between meals—drink one half ounce of liquid per pound of body weight (if you weigh 130 pounds, that's 65 ounces). But no matter how much you weigh, make sure you get a minimum of 64 ounces. Water, green tea, cinnamon-spiced tea, and oolong tea are excellent choices; caffeinated drinks, alcohol, and fruit juices don't count.

BREAKFAST

    3 oz. low-fat sliced ham

    ½ grapefruit, sweetened to taste with stevia

SNACK

    1 small can water-pack tuna

    3 carrot sticks

LUNCH

    Large salad:

       greens, tomato

    3 oz. cooked turkey
    sliced hardboiled egg
  8 oz. skim milk

SNACK

  1 large, fresh apple

DINNER

  6 oz. lean broiled hamburger

  2 slices tomato

  2 large lettuce leaves

  1 T. ketchup

SUPPLEMENTS

- 2 ABC Antioxidant Mixture, twice a day with food
- 2 ABC Warming Herb Mixture, twice a day (Take one hour before eating or two hours after.)
- 3 ABC Warming Amino Mixture, three times a day
- 200 mg SAM-e, twice a day, upon awakening and at midmorning

Exercise

Exercise until you notice that you're sweating, then go eighteen more minutes.

Sleep

Take a short nap if you have to and keep implementing the strategies from weeks 1 and 2 to limit your sleep to a good seven and a half to eight hours.

Day 20

Perspective

I respect my body and keep it healthy.

Lifestyle

Do something crazy. Close your office or bedroom door and dance for a few minutes. The exercise will give you more energy, and, if someone happens to walk in, the embarrassment you'll feel will trigger an even bigger dopamine release.

Diet and Supplements

Throughout the day—with and between meals—drink one half ounce of liquid per pound of body weight (if you weigh 130 pounds, that's 65 ounces). But no matter how much you weigh, make sure you get a minimum of 64 ounces. Water, green tea, cinnamon-spiced tea, and oolong tea are excellent choices; caffeinated drinks, alcohol, and fruit juices don't count.

BREAKFAST

> 1 c. low-fat yogurt
> ¾ c. low-fat cottage cheese
> ½ c. peaches in fruit juice
> 1 T. almonds

SNACK

> Protein shake:
>> whey protein powder, vanilla flavor shake (8 grams of protein)
>> 1 medium banana
>> 1 c. strawberries
>> 2 T. almonds
>> water and ice to taste

LUNCH

> 4.5 oz. grilled chicken breast
> ½ c. chopped broccoli
> 1 c. tossed salad
> 3 T. regular dressing
> 1 small apple

SNACK

> 3 celery stalks stuffed with low-fat cream cheese or peanut butter

DINNER

> 4.5 oz. salmon
> Grilled vegetables:
>> 4 onion slices
>> 1 red pepper

1 zucchini

1 T. dressing for marinade

2 c. tossed salad

SUPPLEMENTS

- 2 ABC Antioxidant Mixture, twice a day with food
- 2 ABC Warming Herb Mixture, twice a day (Take one hour before eating or two hours after.)
- 3 ABC Warming Amino Mixture, three times a day
- 200 mg SAM-e, twice a day, upon awakening and at midmorning

Exercise

Exercise until you notice that you're sweating, then go nineteen more minutes.

Sleep

Take a short nap if you have to and keep implementing the strategies from weeks 1 and 2 to limit your sleep to a good seven and a half to eight hours.

Day 21

Perspective

I have the power to be whoever I want to be.

Lifestyle

Use your feet. Walk or bike someplace you'd normally drive to. Get off the train or bus a stop or two early and use a little shoe leather. Park your car a few blocks away from wherever it is you're going. Pretend your elevator is out of service and take the stairs.

Diet and Supplements

Throughout the day—with and between meals—drink one half ounce of liquid per pound of body weight (if you weigh 130 pounds, that's 65 ounces). But no matter how much you weigh, make sure you get a minimum of 64 ounces. Water, green tea, cinnamon-spiced tea, and oolong tea are excellent choices; caffeinated drinks, alcohol, and fruit juices don't count.

BREAKFAST

    1 c. low-carb cereal

    1 c. skim milk

SNACK

    6 oz. fat-free vanilla yogurt

LUNCH

    Tuna salad:

         5 oz. tuna

         ½ celery stalk, diced

         1 T. onion, diced

         3 T. low-fat mayonnaise

    1 small pickle

    1 medium orange

SNACK

    ¼ c. roasted soy nuts

    ¼ c. golden raisins

DINNER

    6 oz. grilled veal chops

    1 c. red peppers

    1 c. mushrooms

    3 c. spinach

    2 T. low-fat dressing

    ½ c. applesauce

SUPPLEMENTS

- 2 ABC Antioxidant Mixture, twice a day with food
- 2 ABC Warming Herb Mixture, twice a day (Take one hour before eating or two hours after.)
- 3 ABC Warming Amino Mixture, three times a day
- 200 mg SAM-e, twice a day, upon awakening and at midmorning

Exercise

Exercise until you notice that you're sweating, then go twenty more minutes.

Sleep

Take a short nap if you have to and keep implementing the strategies from weeks 1 and 2 to limit your sleep to a good seven and a half to eight hours.

WEEK FOUR

This week's theme is to forget about the past. The only thing you can change about it is how you think about it now. Learn from it and grow. Stay focused on where you are and where you're going instead of where you've been. Forgive yourself.

We're making a few more changes to your supplements and continuing to build stamina by increasing your exercise time one minute a day. If you're still feeling sleepy or lack energy, you must absolutely resist the temptation to use food to keep you awake.

Day 22

Perspective

Today's mission statement is: I have no regrets. I can't change the past, but I can create the future I want.

Lifestyle

Watch bright colors. Dull colors calm us down, but bright ones arouse and stimulate us. Like so many other animals, we humans are naturally attracted to bright colors because they often hold something we need—food.

Diet and Supplements

Throughout the day—with and between meals—drink one half ounce of liquid per pound of body weight (if you weigh 130 pounds, that's 65 ounces). But no matter how much you weigh, make sure you get a minimum of 64 ounces. Water, green tea, cinnamon-spiced tea, and oolong tea are excellent choices; caffeinated drinks, alcohol, and fruit juices don't count.

BREAKFAST

    1 low-carb waffle

    1 sliced banana

    8 oz. low-fat or nonfat milk

SNACK

    2 oz. almonds

LUNCH

    5 oz. low-fat ham

    low-fat mayonnaise, Dijon mustard, lettuce, tomato

    green salad with 1 T. fat-free dressing

    1 small apple

SNACK

    1 medium fresh pear

DINNER

    6 oz. lean roast beef

    2 slices tomato

    2 large lettuce leaves

    1½ T. low-fat mayonnaise

    1 tangerine

SUPPLEMENTS

- 2 ABC Antioxidant Mixture, twice a day with food
- 2 ABC Warming Herb Mixture, twice a day (Take one hour before eating or two hours after.)
- 3 ABC Warming Amino Mixture, three times a day
- 200 mg SAM-e, twice a day, upon awakening and at midmorning

Exercise

Exercise until you notice that you're sweating, then go twenty-one more minutes.

Sleep

Stick with the diet and keep implementing the sleep strategies in weeks 1 to 3. Do everything you can to limit your sleep time to no more than seven and a half to eight hours.

Day 23

Perspective

My goals and desires are clear and reasonable and I know I can accomplish them.

Lifestyle

Ride a roller-coaster. Logically, we know there's nothing to fear, but our brain still perceives a threat and responds accordingly, releasing dopamine and norepinephrine and activating our fight-or-flight response.

Diet and Supplements

Throughout the day—with and between meals—drink one half ounce of liquid per pound of body weight (if you weigh 130 pounds, that's 65 ounces). But no matter how much you weigh, make sure you get a minimum of 64 ounces. Water, green tea, cinnamon-spiced tea, and oolong tea are excellent choices; caffeinated drinks, alcohol, and fruit juices don't count.

BREAKFAST
   2 scrambled eggs
   1 banana

SNACK
   ½ c. roasted soy nuts

LUNCH
   1 medium sweet potato topped with:
         2 oz. shredded jack cheese
         ½ c. broccoli
         ½ c. chopped carrots
   1 c. fresh pineapple chunks

SNACK
   Kiwi smoothie:
         1 medium kiwi, without skin
         4 oz. orange juice
         4 oz. nonfat milk

DINNER

Sauté items with soy sauce to taste:

¾ c. low-fat tofu

1 c. red peppers

1 c. broccoli

1 T. olive oil

1 c. brown rice

2 c. tossed salad

1 T. salad dressing

SUPPLEMENTS

- 2 ABC Antioxidant Mixture, twice a day with food
- 2 ABC Warming Herb Mixture, twice a day (Take one hour before eating or two hours after.)
- 3 ABC Warming Amino Mixture, three times a day
- 200 mg SAM-e, twice a day, upon awakening and at midmorning

Exercise

Exercise until you notice that you're sweating, then go twenty-two more minutes.

Sleep

Stick with the diet and keep implementing the sleep strategies in weeks 1 to 3. Do everything you can to limit your sleep time to no more than seven and a half to eight hours.

Day 24

Perspective

I know that change is important and I welcome every change as an opportunity for growth.

Lifestyle

Read a good book. Reading, even though you probably do it silently, is actually an auditory function—your brain hears the words that your eyes see. Engaging your emotions stimulates dopamine production.

Diet and Supplements

Throughout the day—with and between meals—drink one half ounce of liquid per pound of body weight (if you weigh 130 pounds, that's 65 ounces). But no matter how much you weigh, make sure you get a minimum of 64 ounces. Water, green tea, cinnamon-spiced tea, and oolong tea are excellent choices; caffeinated drinks, alcohol, and fruit juices don't count.

BREAKFAST

    4 whole grain low-carb pancakes

    ½ c. sugar-free fruit compote

    1 c. low-fat milk

SNACK

    Protein shake:

        whey protein powder, vanilla flavor shake (8 grams of protein)

        1 small mango

        1 c. blueberries

        2 T. walnuts

LUNCH

    5 oz. low-fat sliced turkey breast

    2 slices cheddar cheese

    tomato slices, lettuce

    1 c. mandarin oranges

SNACK

    1 T. peanut butter on celery sticks

DINNER

    5 oz. baked scallops

    1 c. chopped lettuce

    4 T. diced tomato

    ½ small diced carrot

    2 T. low-fat dressing

SUPPLEMENTS
- 2 ABC Antioxidant Mixture, twice a day with food
- 2 ABC Warming Herb Mixture, twice a day (Take one hour before eating or two hours after.)
- 3 ABC Warming Amino Mixture, three times a day
- 200 mg SAM-e, twice a day, upon awakening and at midmorning

Exercise

Exercise until you notice that you're sweating, then go twenty-three more minutes.

Sleep

Stick with the diet and keep implementing the sleep strategies in weeks 1 to 3. Do everything you can to limit your sleep time to no more than seven and a half to eight hours.

Day 25

Perspective

Today I will open my mind to the many new opportunities that surround me.

Lifestyle

Take an exercise class at a local health club. By now you've built up some stamina, so instead of your usual exercise routine, do some aerobics. If you can't do it in a club, buy or rent a video and do it at home.

Diet and Supplements

Throughout the day—with and between meals—drink one half ounce of liquid per pound of body weight (if you weigh 130 pounds, that's 65 ounces). But no matter how much you weigh, make sure you get a minimum of 64 ounces. Water, green tea, cinnamon-spiced tea, and oolong tea are excellent choices; caffeinated drinks, alcohol, and fruit juices don't count.

BREAKFAST
  1 scrambled egg

3 strips Canadian bacon

½ grapefruit

1 c. skim milk

SNACK

1 oz. cheese

LUNCH

Chicken Caesar salad:

  4.5 oz. chicken breast

  1 t. grated parmesan cheese

  4 c. red leaf lettuce

  1½ T. Caesar dressing, bottled

20 grapes

SNACK

½ c. roasted pumpkin seeds

DINNER

4.5 oz. grilled halibut

⅔ c. brown rice

10 asparagus spears

2 c. tossed salad

1½ T. low-fat dressing

½ c. fresh or light canned peaches

SUPPLEMENTS

- 2 ABC Antioxidant Mixture, twice a day with food
- 2 ABC Warming Herb Mixture, twice a day (Take one hour before eating or two hours after.)
- 3 ABC Warming Amino Mixture, three times a day
- 200 mg SAM-e, twice a day, upon awakening and at midmorning

Exercise

Exercise until you notice that you're sweating, then go twenty-four more minutes.

Sleep

Stick with the diet and keep implementing the sleep strategies in weeks 1 to 3. Do everything you can to limit your sleep time to no more than seven and a half to eight hours.

Day 26

Perspective

I will keep my eyes on my goals and not let worry and doubt take control of my life.

Lifestyle

Wake up and smell the peppermint. As with strong tastes, peppermint and other powerful odors trigger dopamine release.

Diet and Supplements

Throughout the day—with and between meals—drink one half ounce of liquid per pound of body weight (if you weigh 130 pounds, that's 65 ounces). But no matter how much you weigh, make sure you get a minimum of 64 ounces. Water, green tea, cinnamon-spiced tea, and oolong tea are excellent choices; caffeinated drinks, alcohol, and fruit juices don't count.

BREAKFAST
  ½ cantaloupe
  1 c. low-fat cottage cheese
  1 T. almonds

SNACK
  1 handful of walnuts and almonds

LUNCH
  5 oz. light Jarlsberg cheese
  3 slices tomato
  1 small carrot
  1 small pickle

SNACK
  1 c. fresh strawberries with nonfat whipped cream

Dinner

    5 oz. chicken breast

    2 T. barbecue sauce

    1½ c. coleslaw

    1 c. green beans

    ½ c. fresh or canned apricots in light syrup

Supplements

- 2 ABC Antioxidant Mixture, twice a day with food
- 2 ABC Warming Herb Mixture, twice a day (Take one hour before eating or two hours after.)
- 3 ABC Warming Amino Mixture, three times a day
- 200 mg SAM-e, twice a day, upon awakening and at midmorning

Exercise

Exercise until you notice that you're sweating, then go twenty-five more minutes.

Sleep

Stick with the diet and keep implementing the sleep strategies in weeks 1 to 3. Do everything you can to limit your sleep time to no more than seven and a half to eight hours.

Day 27

Perspective

Today I will learn something new and expand my mind.

Lifestyle

Start your day off with a brisk walk or a few minutes of vigorous stretching. It's a lot better than a second cup of coffee.

Diet and Supplements

Throughout the day—with and between meals—drink one half ounce of liquid per pound of body weight (if you weigh 130 pounds, that's 65 ounces). But no matter how much you weigh, make sure you get a minimum of 64 ounces. Water, green tea, cinnamon-spiced tea, and oolong tea are excellent choices; caffeinated drinks, alcohol, and fruit juices don't count.

BREAKFAST

    Scrambled cheese eggs:

        3 whole eggs and 3 egg whites

        1 oz. cheddar cheese

    1 grapefruit

SNACK

    ½ c. golden raisins

LUNCH

    Turkey salad:

        5 oz. sliced turkey breast

        3 T. diced celery

        2 T. diced carrots

        1½ T. reduced fat mayonnaise

SNACK

    1 large sliced carrot with nonfat ranch dressing

DINNER

    2 tacos wrapped in lettuce leaves: low-fat ground beef, olives, low-fat refried beans, grated cheese, diced lettuce, salsa wrapped in romaine lettuce

    1 ear of corn, steamed

    1 bottle nonalcoholic beer

SUPPLEMENTS

- 2 ABC Antioxidant Mixture, twice a day with food
- 2 ABC Warming Herb Mixture, twice a day (Take one hour before eating or two hours after.)
- 3 ABC Warming Amino Mixture, three times a day
- 200 mg SAM-e, twice a day, upon awakening and at midmorning

Exercise

Exercise until you notice that you're sweating, then go twenty-six more minutes.

Sleep

Stick with the diet and keep implementing the sleep strategies in weeks 1 to 3. Do everything you can to limit your sleep time to no more than seven and a half to eight hours.

Day 28

Perspective

I will concentrate on making progress, not on achieving perfection.

Lifestyle

Imagine. Of all the advice we offer, this may be the best and most effective way to stimulate warming neurotransmitter production. Imagine whatever you like. Imagine things you find interesting or exciting. Imagine the happiest, most exciting times in your life and feel them again. Choose good ones, hold them for as long as you can, and come back to them as often as possible. If you didn't have any or can't remember any, make something up—that's what imagination is all about.

Diet and Supplements

Throughout the day—with and between meals—drink one half ounce of liquid per pound of body weight (if you weigh 130 pounds, that's 65 ounces). But no matter how much you weigh, make sure you get a minimum of 64 ounces. Water, green tea, cinnamon-spiced tea, and oolong tea are excellent choices; caffeinated drinks, alcohol, and fruit juices don't count.

BREAKFAST

> 1 c. slow-cooked oatmeal
>
> 1 c. low-fat milk
>
> 1½ T. diced almonds
>
> 1 t. honey
>
> 1 small apple

SNACK

> 8 oz. protein shake (make 16 oz. in blender and drink 8 oz. now):
>> whey protein powder, vanilla flavor shake (8 grams of protein)
>> 1 medium banana

1 c. strawberries

2 T. almonds

16 oz. water

ice to taste

LUNCH

2 c. stir-fry vegetables (carrots, zucchini, broccoli)

1 c. brown rice

1 peach or plum

SNACK

8 oz. remaining protein shake

DINNER

5 oz. steak

1 c. brown rice

2 c. broccoli

3 c. tossed salad

1 T. low-fat dressing

SUPPLEMENTS

- 2 ABC Antioxidant Mixture, twice a day with food
- 2 ABC Warming Herb Mixture, twice a day (Take one hour before eating or two hours after.)
- 3 ABC Warming Amino Mixture, three times a day
- 200 mg SAM-e, twice a day, upon awakening and at midmorning

Exercise

Exercise until you notice that you're sweating, then go twenty-seven more minutes.

After this, to achieve maximum benefit, you should exercise beyond the sweat point for a minimum of thirty minutes, four days a week. And on non-workout days, try to do something to cause a sweat. This will help get some of the cooling excess out of your body and will make it easier to maintain a proper level of warming neurotransmitters.

Tie your exercise activity to a plan or set of goals and apply them to a reasonable timetable. This will keep you motivated and create a reward or positive feedback system as you go. Most people's intent to exercise regularly is undermined by the lack of defined goals and an inconvenient or impractical routine. Consider goals such as strength, flexibility, weight, and body composition.

When you get beyond the 28-day point, start varying your workout. Perhaps buy a set of tapes such as the Winsor Pilates Method or Tae Bo aerobic boxing to cross-train with weights, calisthenics, and aerobics, and experiment with a variety of other types of activity such as a treadmill, elliptical trainer, or Stairmaster. If you can afford it, think about meeting with a trainer regularly once every four to six weeks to help set realistic goals and create a workout plan.

Sleep

Stick with the diet and keep implementing the sleep strategies in weeks 1 to 3. Do everything you can to limit your sleep time to no more than seven and a half to eight hours.

Maintaining Your Balance

Maintaining your balance and staying away from deficiency isn't difficult if you consciously incorporate these simple, warming-stimulating lifestyle choices on a daily basis.

* Stop smoking. Many warming-deficient people smoke. Stopping is the first and most important thing you can do for your health.
* Start the day off with a boost. Take a shower in the morning rather than at night to get you going, and listen to upbeat talk radio or rhythm-based music like rock 'n' roll rather than classical on your way to work.
* Eat protein frequently through the day.
* Exercise regularly in a way that produces perspiration.
* Make sure you get adequate but not excessive sleep.
* Keep yourself challenged and occupied.
* Drink green tea. Early research shows that the antioxidants found in green tea might inhibit or slow the development of cancer.
* Limit caffeine. One or two coffees or cups of caffeinated tea per day should be your limit. Again, green tea, which has as much or more caffeine than black tea, is preferable because of its antioxidant content.

- Maintaining balance does *not* require any medication. If, however, you feel yourself sliding into a serious deficiency and need medication to keep from completely relapsing, ask your doctor which warming-enhancing drugs would be best for you.
- To maintain healthy NT balance, continue a basic nutritional supplementation program that includes doses of each of the warming antioxidants, herbs, and amino acid supplements specified in the first week of this program.

Make these simple activities part of your daily life. Living in balance, purposely, with a plan and a strategy is not just maintenance: it's prevention.

Working with Your Doctor to Get Back in Balance

Sometimes, despite your best efforts, you may need a little extra help from your doctor to get your dopamine and norepinephrine levels into the proper balance. In these cases your physician may prescribe specialized herbs, hormones, prescription drugs, and even biofeedback. In the following sections we'll talk about how each of these options works and what the potential side effects are. Remember, though, *do not* try any of this except as directed by your physician. Not following his or her directions or making adjustments on your own can be dangerous, if not life-threatening. For those reasons we're not including information on specific dosages. If you're interested in any of the approaches we discuss in this section, consider taking this book along next time you see your doctor.

Hormones

Hormones are natural chemicals produced by the human body. They're responsible for regulating a number of critical organ functions, are involved in cell development and repair, and help modulate our behavior. You can get many hormone precursors (the chemicals that turn into hormones after the brain and body break them down a little), including androstenedione, the precursor for testosterone, without a prescription, but we strongly recommend that you consult with your physician or a trained health care provider *before* taking any of them.

Many psychiatrists are starting to pay attention to the role of hormones in mood and memory disorders including depression, anxiety, and dementia. Three hormones are closely linked with warming neuro-transmitters: human growth hormone (HGH), testosterone, and thyroid. The effects of each on brain chemistry have been studied extensively, and they are sometimes prescribed as part of the treatment for heat deficiency states.

Human Growth Hormone

HGH is a naturally occurring hormone that increases energy and stimulates glutamate production. Most of us are slightly deficient in HGH by the time we're thirty-five or forty, which is why we experience decreases in our drive, motivation, and ability to concentrate. More pronounced deficiencies cause weight gain around the middle and extreme fatigue.

If your physician determines that you're growth-hormone deficient (which requires a special stimulation test), HGH replacement should help you regain your balance. Unfortunately, there are no natural substances or nonprescription items that have been shown to consistently and adequately replenish growth hormone levels.

Dopamine and Testosterone

Testosterone is the hormonal equivalent of dopamine, and many of its effects closely resemble dopamine's. Symptoms of low testosterone include decreased sex drive, erectile dysfunction, muscle weakness, low endurance, and infertility.

Dopamine and testosterone are both major players in the reward centers of the brain, the part of the brain that encourages you to repeat pleasurable activities by giving you a little jolt of dopamine as a reward. Increasing testosterone levels often produces the same results as increasing dopamine, including an increased desire for sex, aggressiveness, and reduced fatigue.

Recent studies have also shown that testosterone acts as a powerful antidepressant, particularly in older men. In one study, thirteen elderly men who reported depression were given testosterone for one month and a placebo for another month. They were not told which month they were receiving which pills. The effects were so clear that twelve of the thirteen subjects were able to correctly identify the month they were taking the testosterone.

As men's testosterone levels decline in midlife, men experience many of the same emotional traumas—particularly depression—women do as their estrogen levels drop. This confirms the theory by other researchers that "male menopause" exists. Men who take testosterone report an increased sex drive, more aggressiveness in business transactions, less irritability, greater happiness, and generally more contentment.

Caution: Take testosterone *only* at the direction of your health care professional—especially if you're male. As testosterone levels rise, the body seeks to maintain balance by converting testosterone into its mirror image, estrogen. This can lead to testicle atrophy and impotence and has been linked to prostate cancer.

Norepinephrine and Thyroid

Thyroid is the hormone most associated with norepinephrine, and its effects are very similar to norepinephrine's. Hypothyroidism (low levels of thyroid) and impairments of *thyroid-related protein* (the protein that transports thyroid in the bloodstream) are clearly linked to major depressive symptoms, which are physical and psychological. Thyroid dysfunction is 20–30 percent more common among people with mood disorders than in the rest of the population. Symptoms of hypothyroidism can be physical as well, leading to extreme fatigue, a puffy look—especially in the eyes—dry hair or hair loss, slow heart rate, and constipation.

Thyroid is often prescribed along with other antidepressants because it increases norepinephrine release and because it also reduces the time it takes for antidepressants to become effective (this can sometimes be as long as a few months).

EEG Biofeedback (Neurofeedback)

Neurofeedback is a technique designed to teach you how to regulate your own brain waves. We're including it in this section because it's a process that you have to be taught, but you generally can't get in to see a biofeedback professional without a physician referral. An electroencephalogram (EEG) measures and quantifies electrical brain wave activity in various parts of the brain. The two brain wave speeds we're concerned with here are slow (*theta*) and fast (*alpha*). Fast brain wave states are associated with concentration and focused thinking, while slow states are associated with mental drifting and attention problems. Slow brain wave states, particularly in the frontal lobes, are also associated with low dopamine—some researchers call this the *lazy frontal lobe syndrome*.

Using a computer that displays detailed EEG information, a trained instructor teaches patients specific techniques to increase their fast brain waves while reducing their slow ones. This results in an increase in brain dopamine production.

Neurofeedback has been used to treat migraines, ADD, ADHD, and many other dopamine and/or norepinephrine-deficit related conditions except those that are caused by actual physical destruction of dopamine neurons (such as Parkinson's disease). Studies have shown that increasing fast brain wave activity can produce clinical improvements in concentration, reduce ADD symptoms, improve mood, and decrease sleep problems. The techniques may take a while to master—sometimes as many as fifty one-hour sessions—but results can be permanent.

Prescription Drugs

Your physician and/or psychiatrist have access to a number of antidepressants and other pharmacological agents that can increase the production and release of dopamine and norepinephrine. As always, even though you may be 100 percent sure that you have a dopamine or norepinephrine deficiency, don't start taking any of these drugs without consulting a trained medical professional familiar with their use. Just because a friend or relative may be taking one of the drugs we discuss below doesn't mean it will work for you.

In addition, some of these drugs work in strange ways, and you want to have your reactions to the drugs monitored by someone who knows what he or she is doing. Some dopamine-enhancing drugs, for example, give some people an irresistible urge to sleep—exactly the opposite of what you'd expect from a neurotransmitter that's generally a stimulant and is used to increase energy levels.

Drugs That Increase Dopamine or Norepinephrine and/or Block Serotonin

Wellbutrin (bupropion)

The most common dopamine-enhancing drug. It works by blocking the "reuptake" of dopamine, meaning that it keeps it from breaking down and disappearing, which has the effect of keeping it working in the brain longer. Most often prescribed as an antidepressant, Wellbutrin has none of the side effects associated with SSRIs (selective serotonin reuptake inhibitors, drugs that work on the inhibitory neurotransmitters), such as fatigue and the inability to reach orgasm. Depending on the circumstance, Wellbutrin is also used by some physicians to increase attention span, stimulate weight loss, increase the sex drive and energy, stop smoking, and overcome a lack of initiative and *anhedonia* (the inability to take pleasure in life). It's also being used to treat ADHD. In weaker concentrations, bupropion is marketed as Zyban, which is used to help alleviate cigarette addiction. Wellbutrin and Zyban have very few side effects, but in high doses they act like stimulants and may cause hypertension, decreased appetite, headaches, and seizures. Caution: Don't take if you have a history of epilepsy or seizures.

Provigil (modafanil)

Also acts to stimulate dopamine production in the brain. It's often prescribed to promote wakefulness, which makes it particularly effective in treating narcolepsy and the fatigue associated with sleep apnea, Parkinson's, and multiple sclerosis. Preliminary studies indicate that Provigil may also be effective as an alternative to stimulants in treating adults with ADD. It may also be effective as an antidepressant, particularly for those who have fatigue and tiredness associated with the SSRIs. Common side effects include headaches and insomnia; taken in excess it can cause euphoria. Caution: Use only under the direction of a physician who has a lot of experience with this drug.

Strattera (Atomoxetine)

The newest drug for ADHD. Because it acts by increasing norepinephrine, it increases alertness and attention and may also be effective as a psychostimulant. Strattera also increases dopamine levels in the frontal lobes of the brain. It has recently been approved by the FDA as a treatment for ADHD. Strattera shows special promise for ADD/ADHD children who have tics and twitches because, unlike many of the alternative drugs, it doesn't aggravate them.

Psychostimulants (Ritalin [methylphenidate], Dexedrine, Cylert, Adderall)

Basically amphetamines or amphetamine-like drugs that temporarily increase the activity of brain cells involved in the stimulus/response process. They act in two ways, stimulating dopamine production and blocking reuptake at the same time. In low dosages, these drugs produce a number of socially desirable effects, such as increased energy and mood, heightened awareness and ability to concentrate, greater self-confidence, more rapid and clearer thoughts, and increased talkativeness and friendliness. They may also act as appetite suppressants. In the short term, psychostimulants have been very successful in helping children with learning disabilities and ADD/ADHD focus and pay attention, and adults or children suffering from extreme fatigue or narcolepsy. Long-term results are harder to determine.

Interestingly, prescription psychostimulants don't always work, which can be frustrating to doctors as well as patients. Recently, however, researchers discovered that there's a far greater chance that the drugs will work if the patient's zinc levels are normal.

Side effects of psychostimulants can include weight loss (which few people complain about), irritability, sleep disturbances, tics, and seizures. Caution: There are two potential problems with psychostimulants. First, there's the "crash effect" when the effect of the drugs wears off, which causes users to want to take more of the drugs more often. Second, when taken in large doses for long periods of time they can lead to amphetamine (or dopamine) psychosis. Symptoms include paranoia, schizophrenia, delusions, hallucinations, aggressive and violent behavior, repetitive and nervous behavior. They can also exaggerate the symptoms of Tourette's syndrome. Don't take any psychostimulant if you've ever suffered from anxiety, heart problems, or drug addiction—or if you're taking any MAO inhibitors (see below) or have taken any within the past fourteen days.

MAO Inhibitors

Block production of *monoamine oxidase,* a chemical that breaks down dopamine in the brain. By inhibiting MAO, these drugs increase the brain's stores of dopamine. *Selegiline* is one of the more common MAOIs. It has been used successfully to slow the progression of Parkinson's disease.

Drugs That Increase Acetylcholine

Acetylcholine's effects are most obvious in the areas of attention and cognition. Drugs that enhance acetylcholine work by blocking *cholinesterase,* the enzyme that normally breaks down acetylcholine, thus leaving more of it in the brain to work. These include the following:

Aricept (donepezil) and Exelon (rivastigamine)

These drugs are typically used to treat Alzheimer's disease and other dementias. Some researchers have begun using these drugs for other conditions, including cognitive and memory impairments related to ADD/ADHD, head injury, stroke, and multiple sclerosis. Side effects include gastric irritation and slowed pulse rate.

Reminyl (galanthamine)

The active ingredient in Reminyl is an alkaloid found in a Chinese medical compound called *shisuan,* which is derived from the common daffodil plant. Reminyl is a stimulant that acts as a *cholinesterase inhibitor* similar to Aricept and Exelon. Reminyl works on a specific set of acetylcholine receptors called *nicotine receptors,* which are located in the pleasure centers of the brain and mediate the relationship between acetylcholine and dopamine. When the nicotine receptors are stimulated they trigger the release of acetylcholine and dopamine. This gives Reminyl a distinct advantage over Aricept and Exelon, both of which work only on acetylcholine. The FDA has recently approved Reminyl as an Alzheimer's treatment. In addition, this drug may be effective in treating ADD, hyperactivity, Tourette's syndrome, autism, and smoking addiction.

Now that you've finished this plan to boost your warming neurotransmitters, we know that you've already begun to see positive changes in your body, mood, behavior, and energy levels. Keep in mind, though, that you're only at the beginning. In order to keep feeling as good as you do now, you need to make the elements of this plan part of your daily life. If you do, you'll not only maintain your current level of balance, but you'll also prevent your problems and symptoms from returning. If you don't, you'll start slipping back toward the way you felt a month or so ago. To stay on track, we suggest that every few months you retake the quiz in chapter 2. The better balanced you are, the more control you have over your mental and physical health and the more satisfying and meaningful your life will be.

CHAPTER 7

Cooling Off

How to Balance Your Cooling Neurotransmitter Deficiency

You are probably reading this chapter because the cooling mechanisms that your brain and body use to soothe you, make you feel safe and comfortable, and help you relax may not be working as well as they should. This may cause you to feel fearful and anxious and may be responsible for some of the habits that have made you feel worse.

That's why we've put together a comprehensive, 28-day program that will help you overcome your cooling neurotransmitter deficit and get your brain and your body back in balance. Based on our experience with thousands of cooling-deficient patients, we know that this plan will enable you to recover from the aches and pains, headaches, back and neck stiffness, infections, rashes, fatigue, excessive weight gain or loss, insomnia, hormonal imbalances, and mood problems such as irritability, anxiety, depression, hostility, and aggression, as well as other symptoms that may have plagued you.

As a cooling-deficient person, you're probably champing at the bit already, anxious to get started, ready to dive in and do everything all at once. *But don't give in to the temptation.* The truth is that once you start the program it'll be relatively easy to increase your cooling neurotransmitter levels, and you'll begin seeing some changes pretty quickly. But those changes won't last if you act impulsively or if you move from one phase of the program to another without giving yourself enough time to make the changes permanent.

The 28-Day Cooling Program has seven basic parts and includes lifestyle changes, dietary modification, physical exercise, specific herbal and vitamin remedies, and even hormonal and pharmacological approaches. Here's a brief overview:

1. *Perspective and worldview.* The first step in implementing this program is to make an honest self-appraisal of your life. Change is not possible unless you clearly understand and appreciate the need for it. There is a Kabbalistic saying that what differentiates humans from other animals is that we walk upright on two legs, while animals walk on four. Having our head above our heart makes it possible for our thoughts and beliefs to flow downward, where they can affect our emotions. Neurologically speaking, there's a lot of truth there. Because of the brain's unique position in regulating and maintaining function throughout the body, starting a self-help program by working on your thoughts and feelings makes a lot of sense.
2. *Sleep.* How long and how well you sleep will have a tremendous impact on every other aspect of your life. You should be able to get at least seven uninterrupted hours of restful sleep every night.
3. *Exercise.* This exercise program addresses the specific needs of people with cooling NT deficits. Cooling-deficient people frequently overexercise as a way of coping with their stress. As a result, they burn out too quickly. For that reason our program is designed to ease you in gradually, allowing your brain to safely step up cooling neurotransmitter production without exhausting itself.
4. *Lifestyle.* In this section we include a number of less-strenuous activities and lifestyle changes you can do on a daily basis to increase your cooling neurotransmitter production.
5. *Diet and supplements.* A cooling deficiency is, by definition, a warming excess, which is a high-energy inflammatory state. To correct a cooling deficiency, the primary focus is on eliminating foods that cause inflammatory reactions. After that the focus is on lean protein and complex carbohydrates.
6. *Maintenance.* Once you've raised your cooling neurotransmitters enough to get your mind and body back in balance, you need to keep them there. We'll show you precisely how to maintain your disposition and keep yourself from falling into a deficiency state again.

7. *Working with your doctor.* If you've given the Cooling Program your best shot for the full twenty-eight days and you still aren't feeling as well as you'd like to, go see your doctor. It's possible that some advanced testing may be required in order to get a better handle on your specific imbalance.

A Note on Timing

Your cooling neurotransmitter levels ebb and flow throughout the day, and they're at their peak in the evening. So take advantage of that extra boost and do as many cooling-NT-increasing things as you can after dinner. If you start too early, your cooling levels won't be high enough and you may lose the energy and motivation to do the things you need to be doing. Generally speaking, increase stimulation during the day and decrease it at night so you can properly recover from your daytime activities.

Of course, you can't do everything in the evenings. Because you need to eat throughout the day, the diet and nutrition section of our plan will tell you what you need to do to get you through the morning and afternoon cooling NT troughs. And hopefully you're getting a good night's sleep. But try to implement as many of the perspective, lifestyle, and exercise steps of the program as late in the day as possible. Doing so will make it easier for your brain to reshape and recondition itself.

Getting Under Way

Keep in mind that none of the steps we're suggesting in this program should negatively interact with each other. However, there's a small risk that they could interact with some medication you're taking, so check with your doctor before you begin the program. Never, ever take any of the prescription medications or hormones we discuss here unless your personal physician specifically instructs you to.

Monitor your progress carefully. It is possible to overdo things, which could result in your cooling deficit becoming an excess. If you find yourself feeling sluggish, lethargic, depressed, or unmotivated, you'll need to slow down a little until those symptoms subside.

Before you actually start the program, we want you to have a firm understanding of what you're going to be doing and why. Here's a detailed look at each of the steps.

Perspective and Worldview

Like everything else in nature, your brain has alternating periods of activity and inactivity. If it weren't for the rest periods, the brain would burn itself out. Cooling-deficient people tend to do too much. If you don't get some down time, you'll snap.

If You Are Cooling Deficient with Anxiety

Because your life is often complex and difficult, you will need frequent pauses to bring your mind and body back into harmony. You must create a zero tolerance for nontruths, hysteria, and exaggerations. Ninety percent of the threatening, negative, and disastrous things you brood about and dread never happen. Winning the lottery might help you feel better, but you have better odds of reducing your anxiety if you can do some triage and manage your reactions. This is a two-step process. Start by learning to recognize when you're anxious and what got you that way. Next, evaluate those factors with the following questions:

- What's bothering me?
- Is what's bothering me real or is it exaggerated?
- Is what's bothering me within my control?
- Is what's bothering me really worth my attention or effort?
- What exactly can I do to change what's bothering me?

Honestly assess your ability to influence or control whatever it is that has caused your anxiety. If it's a legitimate concern and there's something you can do to influence it, take action now. If it's not real or if it's beyond your control, let it go. Remember, all negative anxiety comes from an inherent fear of loss. In order to manage anxiety, you must be absolutely clear and honest in determining exactly what potential losses are at stake.

Pay special attention to your spontaneous language. When you speak in exaggerated, self-critical terms, know that those harsh words are a reflection of internal psychic pressure. Remember why you are doing the things you do and recall your true value and purpose in life. Your reward will be an improved ability to focus, a higher level of energy, and a greater sense of well-being.

Severe anxiety is difficult to treat with natural remedies, but two herbs show promise by increasing brain GABA levels. These include *honokiol* (a natural substance found in traditional Japanese *kampo* formulas used to treat anxiety) and *valerian,* which is often used as a mild sedative (see page 205 for more).

Speak to your doctor. Your anxiety may be warning signs of a more serious, underlying medical condition such as heart disease, lung disease, hormonal problems, and even epilepsy. If those and any other serious conditions can be ruled out, ask your doctor about the prescription drug Gabitril (which increases brain GABA levels) and the SSRIs (which increase serotonin).

Herbs and prescription drugs can help with the symptoms, but they can't cure the environmental causes of your anxiety. For that reason, if your anxiety is chronic or comes and goes regularly, please establish a relationship with a good counselor who makes you feel comfortable.

Banishing Negative Thinking

The most common cause of cooling deficiencies is feeling unsafe in your environment. Worrying, often unnecessarily, can be an hourly event for cooling-deficient people. It not only drains their serotonin, causing anxiety, irritability, and restlessness, but it amplifies the deficiency until there isn't enough serotonin available to deal with life's routine problems. Cooling-deficient people tend toward anxiety and restlessness.

As a cooling-deficient person, you need to concentrate on your personal philosophy and see a strong connection to something bigger and more important than yourself. Worldview does *not* have to be spiritual or religious, although if you're inclined in either of those directions, this is the place for it. So spend a little time thinking about the following questions:

1. What do I want to accomplish in my life and what steps am I taking to get there?
2. What are the obstacles I face, and which ones can I truly influence?
3. What have I done in my life that I can be truly proud of?
4. What are the unique attributes and traits that make me different, special, and valuable to everyone else in the world?
5. What about the other people I meet as I go through life—do they have special insights, skills, or abilities as well? If so, how can I acknowledge and benefit from that?
6. Why is my life important and why should it continue and not end right now?

Your honest answers to these questions will give you a stronger sense of your own and everyone else's uniqueness, importance, and reason for living. They'll also remind you of the many wonderful things you've done and of your value and importance to others. You don't need to do anything with these insights other than remember them. You don't even have to remember them all the time, only when you feel anger, hatred, or malice toward anyone or any living thing, yourself included. If you keep even one positive image about yourself in mind during difficult moments, it will change your life, and that, in turn, will change the lives of everyone you meet.

Take comfort in the fact that when the sun rises each day you have a new chance to be the person you've always wanted to be. You never have to be the man or woman you were yesterday if you truly don't want to.

What it really comes down to is the wisdom of the Serenity Prayer: the wish to have the serenity to accept the things you can't change, the courage to change the things you can change, and the wisdom to know the difference. There's no question that having positive thoughts can have a remarkable impact on your life.

Don't be afraid to get some professional help. As incredibly powerful as positive thinking can be, it can't cure everything. And neither can diet or exercise. Some conditions simply require medical intervention. So if you've tried everything in our 28-day program and you're still not feeling well, get your doctor involved. Don't look at it as a failure on your part. In fact, knowing when to ask for help is a sign of maturity and good mental health.

If You Are Cooling Deficient with High Levels of Stress

You have a tendency to take on too much work and you have a tough time saying no. As a first step, we suggest that you start or maintain talk therapy with a qualified professional so you'll be better able to recognize and maintain your boundaries.

At the same time, you must establish physical, cognitive, and spiritual systems to reduce the stress and tone down the frantic nature of your life. Understand and accept that it is part of your nature to be stressed. If you can get into a routine using the following comprehensive approach, you may be able to diminish and possibly eliminate some of your stress.

- Your physical program should be individualized to best meet your needs, but it might contain gentle but sustained exercise (sweating from muscle activity reduces distress), deep breathing, stretching, or some other means of relaxing and elongating the body. Massage, proper nutrition, and some of the lifestyle adjustments outlined in this chapter will also help.

- Your cognitive system should be your way of minimizing distress as soon as you detect it. Trace your stressors to their emotional origins and learn to evaluate them for what they are. Whether your feelings of stress burst out in an explosive flash or smolder constantly, putting them into perspective will help you extinguish the flame.

- Your spiritual system should help you understand yourself at the most basic and subtle level. Remain open, honest, and curious. Developing a deep, abiding connection with some identity, power, or organization greater than yourself increases focus, concentration, creativity, quality of life, and longevity. Seek to understand before being understood. Be patient yet persistent. Remember that the love and generosity you have for others is based on the love and generosity you have for yourself. You are not likely to become the person you've always wanted to be overnight.

Give yourself a reality check. In order to keep your feelings of uncertainty from draining your cooling neurotransmitters, you must see them for what they truly are: unfounded exaggerations that are largely the product of your imagination. Just think of the way you talk about your life: is your job *really* murder? Are you *really* going to get killed if you don't finish that project on time? Do you *really* have a million things to do today? Sure, they're only expressions, but they get inside your brain and influence your behavior—and your health.

There is a simple, effective technique that you can use every time you feel or hear yourself slipping into a pattern of negative thinking. For this to work, go to a comfortable, quiet place, away from the radio, your computer, your friends, your cat, or any other potential distraction. Think about each of the following questions, one at a time, and listen carefully to your thoughts.

1. What exactly am I afraid of?
2. What is the worst thing that could happen if my fear became a reality?
3. Really and truly, how likely is that to happen?

4. If my fear really is real, is there anything I can do about it?
5. If it's not real, or if I'm not sure, or if there's nothing I can do about it, should I really be worrying about it or beating myself up over it?

If you go through this process slowly, chances are that you'll find that more than half of your negative thoughts are based on imaginary fears. Half of those that are left can't be verified as being real or not. Of the ones that are real, most of them are exaggerated. And of the small number that are true and not exaggerated, most are out of your control anyway.

If You Are Cooling Deficient with Depression

The very first thing to remember—and to tell yourself every single day—is that depression is not a character flaw. It's a disease, just like diabetes or cancer. Just as you would never suggest that someone should feel ashamed or embarrassed because he or she needs insulin or chemotherapy, you shouldn't feel ashamed or embarrassed if you need a little help too.

Still, there are a few things that you can do that may help with your depression before you start taking drugs.

- Exercise. Exercise causes the brain to release *endorphins* (*endoge-nous *morph*ines—in other words, the morphines within us), which are the brain's natural opiates. They're natural pain killers and help regulate and improve our mood. But don't overdo it. Exercising too, as we discuss in this chapter, can overtax your system and leave you feeling worse than before.
- Try some over-the-counter remedies. If your depression is mild, St. John's wort (see page 205) and SAM-e (page 127) are good choices.
- If neither option works, you can make an appointment with a psychiatrist to discuss SSRIs, knowing that you've given it your best shot.

Each week of the program will have a different perspective and worldview theme, and for each day we'll give you a specific mission statement to focus on that will reinforce that theme. Here are several ways you can increase the effectiveness of these mission statements:

- Set aside at least ten minutes every day when you can be quiet and alone. Repeat the statement to yourself several times. Think about it but don't judge it. Add images and visualize what you're saying.

- At night, just before bed, write out the next day's statement and tape it up in places you're likely to go the next morning, such as the bathroom mirror and the refrigerator.
- Make each statement your computer's screen saver for the day.
- Write the statement out ten times, but from several different perspectives: "I am healthy." "She, Jane, is healthy." "You are healthy."

Sleep

Cooling-deficient people typically have some form of sleep-related problems—difficulty falling or staying asleep or getting back to sleep once awakened, teeth grinding, frequent nighttime urination, and sweating. The more cooling-deficient you are, the more numerous and worse these problems will be.

When they are sleeping, cooling-deficient people have faster heart and respiratory rates, higher nighttime body temperatures, more frequent nighttime awakenings, and more involuntary movements than non–cooling-deficient people. They also spend a reduced amount of time in what's called *S* (for synchronized) *sleep*. During this period the brain's and body's metabolic processes slow down, allowing our biological engines to cool. The bottom line is that if you're not getting enough sleep, you're not going to be able to recover from your cooling NT deficit.

The Tryptophan/5-HTP Connection

Although there are a number of natural and over-the-counter sleep aids out there, sometimes all it takes is a dose of tryptophan and a bite or two of a simple carbohydrate to increase cooling NT activity enough to give you the restful sleep you need.

Tryptophan is a naturally occurring amino acid found in most animal proteins and dairy products that is especially high in turkey and cow's milk. Tryptophan is part of the reason for post–holiday meal sleepiness. It is also one of the few amino acids surrounded by controversy and the only one that FDA requires a prescription to buy.

Until the early 1990s, L-tryptophan was a very popular sleep aid, particularly among older people who often develop cooling deficiencies and have trouble sleeping. One of the major suppliers of L-tryptophan was a Japanese amino acid manufacturer. During production, a batch of that company's tryptophan was tainted with bacteria and other substances and somehow made it through quality control and into the United States.

A number of people who bought that particular batch of trypto-phan developed a serious immune reaction called *eosinophilia myalgia,* and several died. The FDA immediately withdrew all tryptophan and tryptophan-containing products. With the manufacturer's help, the FDA was able to identify and remove the single batch source. How-ever, in order to avoid a second incident, the FDA decided to maintain tight control over tryptophan and require the amino acid to be manu-factured and distributed with the same strict standards applied to phar-maceuticals. Today, tryptophan is not available without a doctor's prescription and is sold only in some three hundred "compounding pharmacies" (named for the owners' willingness to "compound" or mix medications and other types of agents and remedies).

Ironically, despite FDA restrictions, the nutritional supplement *5 hydroxy tryptophan* (5-HTP) has been and remains available at health food stores and pharmacies across the country. 5-HTP is the raw material used by brain neurons to manufacture serotonin. The hydroxy form of tryptophan is approximately ten times more potent than the prescription form.

If You Are Cooling-Deficient with Insomnia

Your insomnia may be caused by medication or by emotional, psycho-logical, or physical problems, or simply because you're getting older.

We suggest that you begin dealing with your insomnia by imple-menting the suggestions we give for each day of the 28-day program. If you find that you still can't get the rest you need, take 1 mg melatonin or 100 mg 5-HTP before going to bed.

If you're still having trouble, ask your doctor about GABA-enhanc-ing drugs such as Gabitril, Klonopin, and Ambien.

Norepinephrine and Histamine

In the brain, 5-HTP stimulates the production of serotonin, which in turn stimulates the release of GABA, which helps you fall and stay asleep by calming the neurons that are responsible for wakefulness. The vast majority of sleep problems are caused by one of two warming chemicals: the neurotransmitter norepinephrine and histamine, an inflammatory, stimulatory immune system chemical. Interestingly, GABA is more effective in the presence of norepinephrine than it is in the presence of histamine.

If the sleep method combined with the other aspects of the 28-day plan we present in this chapter doesn't resolve your sleep problems, histamine could be the culprit. If so, you may need an antihistamine to get to sleep.

Diphenhydramine (sold under the brand name Benadryl) is known to cause drowsiness in many people. It does so by counteracting the warming action of histamine on neurons that control wakefulness and vigilance. Start with a 25-mg dose of diphenhydramine with a full glass of water about an hour before bedtime. If you lie down and still cannot fall asleep within fifteen to twenty minutes, try an additional 12.5 mg of diphenhydramine.

Sometimes histamine and norepinephrine work together to keep you awake. People experiencing this combined effect often complain of having persistent or runaway thoughts that prevent them from falling asleep or that leave them feeling as though they never slept even when they actually did.

You may need to experiment with these options for a few nights before you find the dose and combination that works best for you. Don't worry—until you get it right, you can manage your morning fatigue or drowsiness by taking a brisk walk, a cool shower, or, if you absolutely have to, a small cup of coffee.

Nighttime Urination

If you're getting up more than once a night to empty your bladder, you need to drink more liquid during the day and stop four or five hours before bed. Of course, void before lying down and try to keep the lighting in your bathroom area as dim as possible to avoid light stimulation when you do get up.

Exercise

Our central nervous system is divided into two separate systems. The *somatic nervous system* controls the muscles and organs that we can consciously control. And the autonomic nervous system (ANS) controls the organs and systems that, for the most part, we can't control.

The ANS is further divided into two systems, which perfectly parallel our binary neurotransmitters. The *sympathetic nervous system* is warming, assertive, and protective. It's our fight-or-flight mechanism, getting us ready for action, increasing heart rate, blood pressure, and blood flow, dilating the pupils, and expanding the lungs.

The *parasympathetic nervous system* is cooling, recuperative, and restorative. It's concerned with conserving energy and does essentially the opposite of what the sympathetic system does, lowering the heart rate and blood pressure, relaxing, calming, soothing.

Inside the brain, serotonin functions like the parasympathetic system, keeping things under control. So increasing brain levels of serotonin leads to an increase of parasympathetic activity, and doing things that increase parasympathetic activity leads to an increase of serotonin in the brain.

The cooling-deficient person, with an excess of warming neurotransmitters, needs to learn to slow down and take things a little easier. While it's true that exercising is a great way to relax, some cooling-deficient folks go too far, exercising too intensely. The problem is that a cooling deficiency makes it hard to properly regulate one's temperature while working out; some severely deficient people aren't able to perspire. This is potentially self-destructive and can lead to overexertion and exhaustion.

For that reason, the ideal exercise program for the cooling-deficient person is one that stimulates the parasympathetic system while reducing the participation of the sympathetic system. In order to successfully increase your cooling NT levels, you'll have to take a very gradual approach to exercise that allows each day's exertion to gently reassure the body that it can safely allow a little more exertion and heat production.

This means shifting your workout from resistance training and intense exertion to more focused and sustained activities such as stretching, basic calisthenics, and core strengthening. Active, isolated stretching with a partner or workouts utilizing a Swiss ball make excellent fitness routines for the cooling-deficient person, as do various types of exercise that focus on relaxation and breathing such as Pilates, yoga, tai chi, and qigong. You might want to pick up an introductory yoga or stretching tape at your local store or online.

Doing this for twenty-eight days will enable you to achieve balance. And when you get there, you and everyone around you will know it. A balanced person looks and feels relaxed. He or she emanates an aura of confident calm that is reassuring and not arrogant. Following this exercise program will result in unexpected benefits in terms of your physical ability and appearance. Remember that your workouts during these twenty-eight days are not meant to increase your strength or improve your aerobic capacity. Your goal right now is to stretch, extend, and relax. Focus on your breathing and on letting go.

Just to be sure, you should check with your doctor to make sure that this kind of gentle exercise program is okay. If it is, start off easy and be gentle. Your muscles are probably pretty tight and you'll have to gradually coax your body to cooperate. If for some reason this exercise is not okay, we've included at the end of this program a number of less vigorous things you can do to raise your cooling NT levels.

Lifestyle

A critical element of your 28-day plan is to do nothing. Absolutely nothing. A Zen expression says that only after you abandon all thoughts of seeking will you find the path to enlightenment. In other words, you can't have what you want until you no longer want it. While that's a bit of an exaggeration for our purposes, ultimately, doing less is the formula for success for the cooling-deficient person. One of the best ways to do nothing is to make meditation a regular part of your life.

Meditation and Breathing

Meditation is a Sabbath for the brain, an essential period that refreshes and restores, but without the burden of sleep. There are a variety of ways to meditate. You can have a mantra (a word or phrase that you repeat over and over again), you can imagine yourself in a serene setting, you can focus on the sounds in your environment, you can recall in detail the memory of a pleasant or comforting experience, and many others. One thing almost all forms of meditation have in common, though, is that they emphasize breathing. In fact, one of our favorite kinds of meditation—and perhaps the easiest to start with if you're a beginner—is to simply focus on your breath.

Start by going to a quiet, comfortable place. Sitting in a chair or lying on your bed with a pillow under your knees are fine. Then close your eyes and turn your full attention to your breath, concentrating on the air coming in as you inhale and on the air going out as you exhale. Try to take the breath into your belly as opposed to your chest. Simply paying attention to your breath will naturally slow it down, and your brain activity will follow suit.

But be prepared: after about six seconds your mind will start to wander, which is perfectly natural. Once you become aware that this has happened, gently steer your attention away from the distraction and back to your breath. As you breathe, try to prolong the exhalation phase, spending twice as much time exhaling as inhaling. This will lead you into deeper and deeper states of relaxation and will help replenish your cooling neurotransmitters.

Don't Judge Yourself

Perhaps the most important aspect of your meditation is to not judge your performance. We've found that cooling-deficient people often become concerned that they're "doing it wrong." In reality, there's no such thing as meditating wrong.

Just think about some of the times in your life that when you were able to create perfect stillness and peace of mind. Maybe it was when you were doing something as simple as mowing your lawn or watching the sunset. Or maybe it was when you were "in the zone" while swimming, running, or doing some other sport. You experienced a feeling of losing yourself in whatever you were doing. You were so absorbed that you lost track of time and all your worries and concerns—and even the rest of the world—seemed far, far away. You may not have thought of those brief periods as meditation, but that's exactly what they were. So forget about the scoreboard and just do your best.

Meditating is an important part of this program, and you'll be doing it every day. But it isn't the only relaxing way to increase your cooling NT levels. There are a number of things you can do that don't involve very much work at all, and we'll give you one to do every day in addition to your meditation. Two particularly important ones that you can do anytime you want are:

Smell (and taste) the roses.   Researchers have found that our senses of smell and taste—both of which are often related to food—can also have a significant impact on our cooling neurotransmitter levels. The *olfactory bulb* (the part of the brain that processes aromas) is closely linked with the limbic system (the part of the brain the processes emotions) and is known to contain almost all the neurotransmitters that are found elsewhere in the brain.

Certain aromas can produce changes in brain wave activity as well as the release of neurochemicals. Aromas such as lavender and chamomile stimulate the *raphe nucleui* which releases serotonin. Chamomile scent is often used in aromatherapy as a calming agent and to treat depression. Lavender has been used to treat insomnia. It contains *oxygenated terpenes,* which interact with cell membranes to suppress cell movement and create a sedative effect.

Listen up.   As with scent, we seem to have an intuitive understanding of how sound affects us. People are often described as upbeat or marching to the beat of a different drummer.

Music and sounds stimulate both sides of our brain but in different ways, according to Joshua Leeds, author of *The Power of Sound.* Harmony, rhythm, and low pitches, for example, stimulate a serotonin release, which calms and relaxes us. Atonality, fast rhythms, and high-pitched noise and instruments tend to excite and agitate, stimulating the dopamine system.

If we skip the assumption that certain pieces of music are inherently likable while others are not, it's safe to say that music that increases a person's serotonin meets that person's need to increase cooling NTs.

If You Are Cooling Deficient with Recurrent Headaches

A headache every once in a while is usually nothing to worry about. But if you're having regular or frequent headaches, you should see your doctor. Although serious causes of headaches are uncommon, early detection if there is a problem can be lifesaving. Some other things that may help reduce your headaches are listed below.

Watch out for the over-the-counter drugs.   If you're treating your recurring headaches with medication such as Tylenol or Motrin, you may be doing yourself more harm than good. Taken on a regular basis, these drugs can lead to a condition called *rebound hyperalgesia,* which depletes serotonin and may even cause headaches—exactly the opposite effect from what you were hoping to accomplish.

Eliminate all caffeine products.   Although caffeine is one of the active ingredients in many migraine medications, caffeine withdrawal can cause headaches of its own.

Try some magnesium.   Magnesium increases GABA in the brain and reduces the blood vessel spasms associated with many kinds of headaches. Start with 200–400 mg per day and be patient—it may take as long as four weeks to get any significant benefit.

Investigate low-dose antidepressants.   If none of these alternatives work, ask your doctor about a low dose of antidepressants or GABA-enhancing drugs such as Depakote, which are very effective in preventing headaches.

Diet

Chances are that when you're feeling your best you're a meat-and-potatoes person because meat increases warming NTs and potatoes increase cooling NTs. But in your current cooling-deficient state, you may have been eating more bread, baked goods, and starchy sweets like cookies than ever before, which reflects your brain's attempt to increase cooling NT activity.

The cooling increasing diet involves several important steps:

1. Monitor your protein intake.   Although you need plenty of protein to keep healthy and to repair and grow your muscles, a very high-protein diet tends to increase warming neurotransmitter levels (and decreases the relative levels of cooling NTs), which is exactly the opposite of what you're trying to do. So eat no more than one serving a day of proteins such as eggs, red meat, and cheese.

    Be sure that the protein you eat is high in tryptophan and relatively low in fat. High-tryptophan, low-fat proteins include skinless chicken and turkey, nuts (especially almonds, cashews, and peanuts), sunflower seeds, legumes, egg whites, skim milk, and low-fat yogurt.

2. Eat plenty of complex carbohydrates.   This includes pasta, potatoes, rice, and whole grain breads, unless you've found out that these foods cause an antibody reaction. These foods trigger insulin release, make tryptophan the most important amino acid in your bloodstream, and relax you. (That glass of warm milk you have to help you get to sleep works by giving you a little dose of lactose, which is a high-carbohydrate milk sugar.) But be careful, because too many carbohydrates can sap your energy completely. If you find that happening, you can counteract the soporific effect by adding some dopamine-enhancing protein to your meal.

3. Eat a lot of fruits and vegetables, particularly ones that are leafy and dark green.   They contain a wonderful mix of vitamins and minerals that help your body process protein and carbs more efficiently. Because fruits and vegetables generally have a high water content, they have a tendency to cool your body—precisely what you need to do if you're in a serotonin-deficient state.

4. Don't forget about fat.   Although we generally advocate a low-fat diet, we never suggest a *no*-fat one. You need fat to survive. In fact, a large percentage of brain receptors are made from fats, and the amount of fat in your diet has a direct impact on the responsiveness

of those receptors. Just make sure you get the right kind: essential fatty acids, which are mostly polyunsaturated fats, such as those from almonds, walnuts, olive oil, and omega-3 and omega-6 fats that come from cold-water fish. The National Institute of Alcohol Abuse in a recent study of dietary habits found a direct relationship between levels of polyunsaturated fatty acids and serotonin levels as measured in cerebrospinal fluid. This means that the more essential fatty acids you consume, the more serotonin your body makes, and vice versa.

The wrong kind of fat—particularly saturated fats and trans fats (hydrogenated or partially hydrogenated oils)—reduces brain cell responsiveness to all neurotransmitters, which results in fatigue and sluggish thinking and can reduce blood circulation by causing blood cells to clump together. In the presence of norepinephrine (which increases when you eat protein), saturated fats become unstable, causing a condition called *oxidative stress,* which in turn produces free radicals, which are responsible for causing tissue and organ damage. The higher the level of saturated fats, the higher the levels of cooling NTs and the less the brain responds to warming ones.

5. Don't go overboard.   As with everything else in our body and our universe, fats aren't all good or all bad, and even the "good" essential fats have better and worse components. Omega-6 fatty acids come largely from egg yolk and fatty meats. And while there's nothing wrong with omega-6 acids in moderation, it's their relative balance with omega-3 acids that can cause problems. The normal ratio of omega-6 to omega-3 should be 1 to 2 (half as much omega-6 as omega-3). The average Western diet, however, is completely out of whack at 25 to 1.

The cure? Get a *lot* more omega-3 in your diet. The heating/cooling metaphor works beautifully here: omega-3 comes mostly from cold-water fish, so taking more of it is like throwing cold water on an overheated brain.

A Note on Cholesterol

It's always a good idea to watch your cholesterol intake, but, as with fats, don't go overboard in either direction. High-cholesterol diets have been associated with reduced aggression. Cholesterol makes more serotonin available in the nerve synapses and stabilizes serotonin transporter molecules, which has the effect of increasing information flow within the brain. When cholesterol levels get too low, there aren't enough transporters to get serotonin where it needs to be. Too much cholesterol can lead to some of the same problems as too much saturated fats—increased risk of blood clots, heart attack, and so on.

At the same time, too little cholesterol isn't good for you either. One fascinating study tracked 50,000 subjects for several years and found that people with very low cholesterol levels—under 160—had three times more injuries than people with more normal levels. In addition, although their risk of heart attack was lower, the low-cholesterol group had a much higher risk of committing suicide than the normal-cholesterol controls.

With the assistance of a colleague, nutritionist Carl Germano, RD, CNS, CDN, we've included a complete 28-day meal plan as part of the Cooling Program. The diet in this chapter provides 1,700 calories per day. However, your caloric requirements may be somewhat different. To determine yours, do one of the following:

1. If you're a woman, multiply your weight in pounds by 12 if you're inactive, 13 if you do light work or exercise, 14 if you do light or moderate work or exercise, 15 for moderate to heavy work or exercise, and 16 for heavy work or exercise.
2. If you are a man, multiply your weight in pounds by 13 if you're inactive, 14 for light work or exercise, 15 for light to moderate work or exercise, 16.5 for moderate to heavy work or exercise, and 18 for heavy work or exercise.

If you have any specific concerns, we suggest that you seek guidance from a registered, certified, or licensed nutritionist.

Keep in mind that although this diet will have an immediate impact on your serotonin levels, the effects generally won't last too long. That means that it will take more than just changing the way you eat to produce any long-term impact on your life.

Dietary Supplements

As already noted, the most fundamental thing you can do to rebalance your neurotransmitters is balance your daily diet. But chances are you'll need more serotonin and/or GABA than you can ingest by eating normally. In this case you may need to take some nutritional supplements, such as herbs, vitamins, and amino acids. All of these are available over the counter in health food stores and drugstores. While most are safe, we'll point out the ones that you should discuss with your physician before taking.

Herbs

Several herbs have been studied and shown to be effective in treating a variety of serotonin-deficit symptoms. Although the two herbs we discuss below are widely available, we can't recommend either with complete confidence. The main problem is that there is little or no standardization in the dietary supplement industry, and it's almost impossible to ensure adequate purity or that the herb you buy provides an appropriate amount of the active ingredient to be effective—regardless of what's printed on the label. Nevertheless, it's worth taking a few minutes to consider them. Although these and other herbs are generally available over the counter, be sure to check with your doctor before taking them. There may be significant negative interactions between certain herbs and other medications you may be taking. Taken under the supervision of a medical professional, these herbs can be extremely effective. Used inappropriately, they can be extremely dangerous.

St. John's wort is the most widely publicized over-the-counter treatment for depression. There's plenty of anecdotal evidence that it works, and a number of studies have been done that confirm that St. John's wort is more effective than placebo. There have also been a number of other studies that show that it doesn't work at all. Until now, the problem has been that each study analyzes a different form of the herb. Most of them also don't define depression or use consistent criteria to determine success or failure. St. John's wort (supposedly) works by inhibiting the reuptake of serotonin. One thing that is known for sure is that there can be dangerous interactions between St. John's wort and a number of other drugs. It lowers the effect of coumadin (an anticoagulant) and some HIV drugs. If you're interested in giving it a try, be absolutely sure to check with your doctor first. Make sure you buy it from a reliable manufacturer and that it contains enough *hypericum* to be effective. Common side effects include nausea, heartburn, and phototoxic rash (getting easily sunburned).

Valerian is used in traditional medicine as a mild sedative and sleep-inducing agent. It works by inhibiting the breakdown of GABA as well as blocking its reuptake. It has a mechanism similar to that of a drug called Gabitril. The roots of valerian contain a complex chemical mixture called *valepotriates,* which have sedative and tranquilizing properties. The problem is that those properties are largely lost in the process of drying the herb. As with St. John's wort, there are considerable problems with standardization, purity, and effectiveness, but it's safe to use on a trial basis (assuming your doctor agrees).

Vitamins and Other Nutritional Compounds

Folic acid is being studied as a supplemental treatment for major depression. Some studies suggest a link between folic acid deficiency and impaired metabolism of serotonin. Low or deficient folic acid levels have been detected in up to 38 percent of depressed adults. Patients with low levels of folic acid are less responsive to SSRIs than those with adequate levels. Even those who aren't folic acid deficient report that SSRIs are more effective when taken with folic acid. In any case, folic acid should be taken with vitamins C and B-12.

Vitamin B-6, also called pyridoxine, is a B vitamin involved in a wide range of biochemical activity including the synthesis of GABA and serotonin. B-6 deficiency leads to increased risk of seizure activity in infants and adults. It leads to irritability and nervousness. B-6 is generally safe to take in doses less than 200 mg per day.

DHA (docosohexanoic acid), also known as "fish oil." This valuable nutrient is another form of omega-3 fatty acids derived from cold-water fish such as salmon and mackerel. DHA reduces inflammation by shifting immune system activity away from the production of inflammatory cytokines (which happens a lot to cooling-deficient people). DHA supplements come in 50- to 120-mg capsules. Taking 10 grams a day (1,000 mg = 1 gram) in combination with magnesium has been shown to effectively reduce elevated blood pressure. One problem associated with taking 10 grams daily is bowel tolerance. Unless you introduce the DHA gradually or augment the DHA with digestive enzymes containing high amounts of lipase, taking anything over 5 grams a day will cause diarrhea. Taking 2 to 4 grams a day can help reduce inflammation, increase healing, and help maintain brain function. Before buying DHA, read the label and other packaging material carefully. Do not buy a product that does not guarantee that the oil contains no mercury and that it is 99 percent pure and nonrancid. If you can't find that information on the package, ask the nearest pharmacist to recommend an appropriate, quality-assured brand.

EPA (eicosapentaenoic acid) is one of the omega-3 fatty acids in which our traditional Western diet is lacking. Patients with clinical depression have been shown to have low blood levels of EPA. And a recent study published in the *Archives of General Psychiatry* reported that one gram per day of ethyl EPA significantly reduced symptoms of depression in a double-blind study.

Myoinositol is a natural compound found in legumes and cereals. It may possess some antidepressant and antianxiety activities, but research is far from conclusive.

Inositol is the active amino acid part of myoinositol. It can greatly increase GABA activity, particularly when taken in an effervescent, buffered form.

Magnesium is an essential mineral, meaning you need to get it through food because your body can't produce enough of it on its own. It's involved in the electrical stability of cells and has been called nature's physiological calcium channel blocker because it reduces the flow of calcium into cells. Magnesium increases the sensitivity of GABA receptors and lowers glutamate sensitivity in the brain. (Note that there's a lot of difference between brain levels and blood levels. In the blood, magnesium actually helps synthesize calcium, which is why you almost always see the two together when you buy calcium supplements.) Elevated warming NT levels cause you to excrete large amounts of magnesium. Magnesium deficiency may lead to muscle cramps, migraines, irregular heart rate, and an increased risk of heart attack and stroke. We recommend 400 to 600 mg per day—more if you can take it without developing diarrhea. The best way to determine your tolerance is to start at about 300 mg per day and increase your dose by 200 mg each day until you have diarrhea, then back off 200 mg. That will allow you to take the maximum dose you can handle without this adverse effect.

Amino Acids

Amino acids are the basic building blocks of just about everything in the body. They're involved in making cells, repairing tissue, and helping the body fight infection. They build proteins and carry oxygen through the body. They're also a common nutritional supplement that you can get at a health food or drugstore near you. They come in two types: the *nonessential* variety are the ones your body can manufacture from other chemicals already in your system; as with minerals, *essential* amino acids can't be manufactured internally and have to be brought into the body via food or supplements. The major amino acid involved in cooling neurotransmitters is tryptophan. One of its natural by-products, 5-HTP, which is what tryptophan becomes before it converts to serotonin, is widely available over the counter.

5-HTP is found mainly in an African plant called *griffonia*, which is a relative of carob. Small amounts are also found in bananas, plums, avocados, eggplant, walnut, and pineapple. It is often recommended as an antidepressant. Some studies have indicated a usefulness in treating insomnia and fibromyalgia.

Putting It All Together:
The 28-Day Cooling Program

Rule 1 for the cooling-deficient person is accept yourself, and that's the theme for this week. No matter what you did or did not do, no matter what was done or not done to or for you, you must acknowledge and accept it and let it go. Accept yourself as you are, no matter what. And for goodness' sake, learn to accept compliments. Accepting compliments is a public display of self love. It is you honoring yourself by welcoming someone else's praise and admiration for you. One way to get better at accepting compliments is to smile as big and open-mouthed as you can every time you sense a compliment coming on. Doing that demonstrates your appreciation for what the other person is saying and makes it easier for him or her to say it. It also makes it easier for you to accept it.

When it comes to sleep, your goal is to get at least seven and a half hours of relatively uninterrupted rest every night. This week you'll start working on achieving that goal by gradually introducing what's called *sleep hygiene*—creating an environment that's more relaxing and conducive to sleep. If you find yourself getting up in the middle of the night, try the suggestions in "Getting Back to Sleep" on page 211. On the other hand, if you snore loudly, sweat profusely, or awaken with a choking sensation, or any painful symptoms occur, make an appointment and consult your doctor immediately. These symptoms require more attention and assistance than you can safely do on your own.

This week you'll be starting an exercise program that will gradually restore your cooling neurotransmitters to a state of balance. Focus on light stretching or exercises that stress relaxation and breathing, such as Pilates, yoga, tai chi, and qigong. If you're already in good shape and work out regularly, do these exercises in addition to your regular workout.

This week we introduce two combinations that will be the foundation of your nutritional supplement program for the rest of the 28-day program. These are:

- The Advanced Brain Chemistry (ABC) Cooling Vitamin Mixture, which consists of
  - 400 mcg folate
  - 50 mg B-6
  - 250 mg inositol
  - 200 mg magnesium
- The cooling supplements, which is not a mixture but comprises separate supplements (we will give specific usage guidelines in the 28-day plans):
  - 100 mg 5-HTP
  - 300 mg EPA twice a day
  - 200 mg DHA twice a day
  - 30 mg 5-HTP in sublingual pearls (widely available) as needed

WEEK ONE

Day 1

Perspective

Today's mission statement is: I accept and love myself the way I am. I don't need anyone else to tell me how to look or feel.

Sleep

Get rid of some vices. Quit smoking—smokers often wake up very early in the morning because of nighttime nicotine withdrawal. Avoid caffeine, a known stimulant, within two hours of bedtime. And keep alcohol consumption to a minimum. One drink a night is fine (as long as your doctor agrees) and may help you sleep. But more than that can interfere with your sleep by increasing wakefulness in the latter half of the evening.

Exercise

Do ten minutes of light stretching in the morning and twenty minutes in the evening not less than ninety minutes before going to bed.

Lifestyle

During the day, find the time to take some long, slow, deep breaths. Although we don't usually pay much attention to our breathing, doing so can actually have a huge impact on our brain and body function. As a general rule, inhalation activates and warms, while exhalation quiets and cools. Animal EEG studies show that when cats and other mammals breathe in, nerve cells across the brain increase their rate of firing, just as adding oxygen to a fire makes it burn harder. Conversely, exhaling slows neural firing. Breathing out more slowly calms our nervous system, particularly the *vagus nerve,* which is the predominant mediator of the parasympathetic (relaxing) system. It also increases the amount of inhibitory, cooling neurotransmitters such as GABA in the brain. It's no wonder, then, that so many meditative traditions—which emphasize prolonging exhalation—produce a sense of peace, relaxation, and inner calm. In the evening, do ten minutes of meditation not less than ninety minutes before bedtime.

Diet and Supplements

You should be drinking liquid with and between meals, throughout the day. Drink half an ounce of liquid per pound of body weight (if you weigh 130 pounds, that's 65 ounces). But whatever your weight, make sure you get at least 64 ounces every day. Water (with or without lemon) and calming herbal teas such as chamomile, white, or valerian teas are fine, but caffeinated drinks, alcohol, and fruit juices don't count.

BREAKFAST
> 1 scoop of whey protein (16 g) mixed with:
>> 1 c. low-fat yogurt with fruit
>> 1 oat bran muffin
>> ½ banana

LUNCH
> 1 Boca burger
> 1 whole wheat bun
> 2 c. brown rice
> 1½ c. tomato
> 1 T. low-fat dressing

DINNER
> 2 c. penne pasta tossed with 1 c. sautéed red peppers and garlic in 1 T. olive oil
> 2 c. tossed green salad with 1 T. low-fat dressing

2 whole grain breadsticks

½ cantaloupe

SUPPLEMENTS

Today take:

- 2 ABC Cooling Vitamin Mixture with breakfast
- 100 mg 5-HTP one hour after dinner
- 300 mg EPA three times a day with food
- 200 mg DHA three times a day with food
- 30 mg 5-HTP in sublingual pearls (available at natural product stores and placed under the tongue). Take as needed throughout the day for calming and cooling.

Getting Back to Sleep

In the first week of the plan, bake a few medium-sized white or sweet potatoes, cut them in thirds, and put them in your refrigerator. An hour before you want to go to sleep, take 50 to 100 mg of 5-HTP. Thirty minutes later, eat a third of one of the potatoes. The starch in the potato will help the 5-HTP get to your brain more effectively. If you don't like potatoes or are allergic to them, eat a rice cake instead. This should help you get to sleep. If you wake up in the middle of the night and can't get back to sleep, eat another third of a potato and take another 50 to 100 mg of 5-HTP with a glass of warm water.

Day 2

Perspective

I accept my imperfections and I will reward myself for my efforts to achieve.

Sleep

Make your bedroom a noise- and light-free zone. Turn off the television, cell phone, and any other distractions. Take your computer out of your bedroom altogether. If you have a watch that chimes every hour, turn that off too. And if you share a bed with someone who snores, get yourself some earplugs.

Exercise

Continue doing ten minutes of relaxing stretching or light exercise in the morning and twenty more in the evening. Buy a stretching or yoga video that has beginner, intermediate, and advanced workouts, and do the one that's right for you.

Lifestyle

Get up a little early and start your day off with a warm, relaxing bath. In the evening, do ten minutes of meditation at least ninety minutes before bedtime.

Diet and Supplements

You should be drinking liquid with and between meals, throughout the day. Drink half an ounce of liquid per pound of body weight (if you weigh 130 pounds, that's 65 ounces). But whatever your weight, make sure you get at least 64 ounces every day. Water (with or without lemon) and calming herbal teas such as chamomile, white, or valerian teas are fine, but caffeinated drinks, alcohol, and fruit juices don't count.

BREAKFAST

　　4 egg whites, scrambled

　　2 slices whole grain toast

　　1 c. fresh berries

　　1 T. Smart Balance spread

LUNCH

　　4 oz. cheese blintzes

　　2 slices pineapple

　　1 c. tossed salad with 1 c. chickpeas

　　1½ T. low-fat dressing

DINNER

　　4 oz. top sirloin, lean

　　1 medium baked potato

　　1½ c. broccoli

　　3 oz. red wine or 2 pineapple slices

SUPPLEMENTS

- 2 ABC Cooling Vitamin Mixture with breakfast
- 100 mg 5-HTP one hour after dinner
- 300 mg EPA three times a day with food

- 200 mg DHA three times a day with food
- 30 mg 5-HTP in sublingual pearls. Take as needed throughout the day for calming and cooling.

Day 3

Perspective

I am a good person even though I sometimes feel angry.

Sleep

Get comfortable. Ideally, your bedroom temperature should be between 65 and 70 degrees Fahrenheit. Too high and you'll get less deep sleep, dream less, and wake up restless. Also, don't eat less than ninety minutes before bedtime. If your digestive system is in full gear, you won't be able to get to sleep as easily.

Exercise

Continue doing ten minutes of relaxing stretching or light exercise in the morning and twenty more in the evening.

Lifestyle

During the day, take some time to read something inspirational—it could be the Bible, it could be the autobiography of someone you admire. In the evening, do ten minutes of meditation at least ninety minutes before bedtime.

Diet and Supplements

You should be drinking liquid with and between meals, throughout the day. Drink half an ounce of liquid per pound of body weight (if you weigh 130 pounds, that's 65 ounces). But whatever your weight, make sure you get at least 64 ounces every day. Water (with or without lemon) and calming herbal teas such as chamomile, white, or valerian teas are fine, but caffeinated drinks, alcohol, and fruit juices don't count.

BREAKFAST

    2 whole grain pancakes

    2 T. fruit preserves

    1 apple

LUNCH

> Tuna pita pocket:
> > 4 oz. water-pack tuna
> > ½ c. tomato, celery, and onion, diced
> > 1 T. low-fat mayonnaise
> > 1 whole wheat pita pocket
>
> 1 c. tossed green salad
>
> 1 T. low-fat dressing
>
> 10 green or purple grapes

DINNER

> 4 oz. baked chicken breast marinated in 3 T. teriyaki sauce
>
> 1 c. snow peas
>
> 1½ c. brown rice
>
> 1 c. tossed green salad with 1 T. low-fat dressing

SUPPLEMENTS

- 2 ABC Cooling Vitamin Mixture with breakfast
- 100 mg 5-HTP one hour after dinner
- 300 mg EPA three times a day with food
- 200 mg DHA three times a day with food
- 30 mg 5-HTP in sublingual pearls. Take as needed throughout the day for calming and cooling.

Day 4

Perspective

I will be accepting of others and more tolerant of their differences.

Sleep

Get the right equipment. If you clench or grind your teeth at night, get a properly fitted bite guard.

Exercise

Continue doing ten minutes of light stretching in the morning and twenty more at night. When stretching, don't bounce up and down. Simply pull and breathe out. Before inhaling, take up the slack—however minute. Now repeat the process, taking up the slack with every exhalation. After fifteen or twenty breaths you'll be amazed at the increase in your range of motion.

Lifestyle

Pack yourself a bag lunch and eat it in a quiet park. In the evening, do ten minutes of meditation at least ninety minutes before bedtime.

Diet and Supplements

You should be drinking liquid with and between meals, throughout the day. Drink half an ounce of liquid per pound of body weight (if you weigh 130 pounds, that's 65 ounces). But whatever your weight, make sure you get at least 64 ounces every day. Water (with or without lemon) and calming herbal teas such as chamomile, white, or valerian teas are fine, but caffeinated drinks, alcohol, and fruit juices don't count.

BREAKFAST

- ½ c. slow-cooked oatmeal, sweetened to taste with cinnamon and/or stevia
- ½ c. nonfat milk
- 1 scoop soy protein powder (16 g)
- 1 T. raisins
- 2 slices whole grain toast
- 1 T. preserves of your choice
- 1 apple

LUNCH

Grilled cheese sandwich:
- 2½ oz. low-fat cheddar or American cheese
- 2 slices whole wheat or whole grain bread
- 1 T. Smart Balance spread or 1 T. spicy mustard

2 carrots sliced into sticks

DINNER

- 4 oz. grilled salmon
- 1 c. sliced tomatoes with 1 T. olive oil, salt, garlic powder, and lemon
- 2 T. low-fat dressing
- 2 c. couscous

2 whole grain breadsticks

1 c. blueberries

SUPPLEMENTS

- 2 ABC Cooling Vitamin Mixture with breakfast
- 100 mg 5-HTP one hour after dinner
- 300 mg EPA three times a day with food
- 200 mg DHA three times a day with food
- 30 mg 5-HTP in sublingual pearls. Take as needed throughout the day for calming and cooling.

Day 5

Perspective

I speak to myself in a loving and supportive way.

Sleep

Go to bed earlier. Every hour of sleep before midnight is worth two after. And avoid daytime naps. They may feel good at the time, but they'll interfere with your nighttime sleep.

Exercise

Continue doing ten minutes of relaxing stretching or light exercise in the morning and twenty more in the evening.

Lifestyle

Cook a delicious dinner for your spouse (or yourself if you live alone) and eat it by candlelight. Do ten minutes of meditation at least ninety minutes before bedtime.

Diet and Supplements

You should be drinking liquid with and between meals, throughout the day. Drink half an ounce of liquid per pound of body weight (if you weigh 130 pounds, that's 65 ounces). But whatever your weight, make sure you get at least 64 ounces every day. Water (with or without lemon) and calming herbal teas such as chamomile, white, or valerian teas are fine, but caffeinated drinks, alcohol, and fruit juices don't count.

BREAKFAST
>   2 slices egg white French toast
>
>   1 sliced banana or 2 T. fruit preserves
>
>   1 c. low-fat yogurt

LUNCH
>   5 oz. turkey breast
>
>   2 slices whole grain toast
>
>   2 T. low-fat mayonnaise
>
>   1 sliced tomato
>
>   3 celery sticks
>
>   1 apple

DINNER
>   1 large grilled pork chop, trimmed of all visible fat
>
>   2 c. basmati rice with peas
>
>   1 c. tossed green salad with 2 T. low-fat dressing
>
>   1 whole grain dinner roll
>
>   ½ c. mandarin oranges in light syrup

SUPPLEMENTS
- 2 ABC Cooling Vitamin Mixture with breakfast
- 100 mg 5-HTP one hour after dinner
- 300 mg EPA three times a day with food
- 200 mg DHA three times a day with food
- 30 mg 5-HTP in sublingual pearls. Take as needed throughout the day for calming and cooling.

Day 6

Perspective

I accept myself as I am now.

Sleep

Go to bed only when you're tired. With the exception of sex, your bed should be used only for sleep. No watching television, no reading, no eating, no folding laundry, no arguing.

Exercise

Continue doing ten minutes of relaxing stretching or light exercise in the morning and twenty more in the evening. Today, instead of getting together with your colleagues in a conference room, take a walk with them and have your meeting on the go.

Lifestyle

Do something that makes you laugh, whether it's watching a funny movie or sitcom, reading a humor book, or going to see a favorite comedian. In the evening, do ten minutes of meditation at least ninety minutes before bedtime.

Diet and Supplements

You should be drinking liquid with and between meals, throughout the day. Drink half an ounce of liquid per pound of body weight (if you weigh 130 pounds, that's 65 ounces). But whatever your weight, make sure you get at least 64 ounces every day. Water (with or without lemon) and calming herbal teas such as chamomile, white, or valerian teas are fine, but caffeinated drinks, alcohol, and fruit juices don't count.

BREAKFAST
   ½ cantaloupe
   1 c. low-fat cottage cheese
   2 small low-fat raisin bran muffins

LUNCH
   5 oz. tuna (water-pack)
   2 T. low-fat dressing
   1 c. diced carrots and celery
   2 slices whole grain toast
   1 c. tossed salad
   1 T. dressing
   1 pear

DINNER
   1½ c. lentil soup
   2 c. chickpea salad with chopped tomato, red pepper, garlic, balsamic dressing

1 c. brown rice

1 c. tossed salad with 2 T. low-fat dressing

1 c. sliced peaches

SUPPLEMENTS

- 2 ABC Cooling Vitamin Mixture with breakfast
- 100 mg 5-HTP one hour after dinner
- 300 mg EPA three times a day with food
- 200 mg DHA three times a day with food
- 30 mg 5-HTP in sublingual pearls. Take as needed throughout the day for calming and cooling.

Day 7

Perspective

I will not worry about what I don't have; I will focus on what I have.

Sleep

Stay away from over-the-counter sleep remedies. They may help you out at first, but you could develop a tolerance, which will aggravate your cooling deficiency and make your sleep problems even worse.

Exercise

Continue doing ten minutes of relaxing stretching or light exercise in the morning and twenty more in the evening.

Lifestyle

Take a news holiday. Consciously avoid listening to the news, watching it on television, talking about it, or even sneaking a peek at newspaper headlines. In the evening, do ten minutes of meditation at least ninety minutes before bedtime.

Diet and Supplements

You should be drinking liquid with and between meals, throughout the day. Drink half an ounce of liquid per pound of body weight (if you weigh 130 pounds, that's 65 ounces). But whatever your weight, make sure you get at least 64 ounces every day. Water (with or without lemon) and calming herbal teas such as chamomile, white, or valerian teas are fine, but caffeinated drinks, alcohol, and fruit juices don't count.

BREAKFAST

  1 c. cold cereal

  1 c. low-fat milk

  1 c. fresh berries

  1 slice whole grain toast with preserves

LUNCH

  1 c. tomato-basil soup

  ½ whole wheat pita pocket stuffed with 2 slices low-fat mozzarella cheese toasted in the oven to melt the cheese

  1 c. tossed green salad with lemon juice to taste, ½ T. olive oil, salt, and pepper if desired

  ½ c. fresh peaches, sliced

DINNER

  5 oz. grilled tilapia fish

  1 c. oven-baked french fries

  2 oven-baked hush puppies

  1 c. green salad tossed with 1 T. low-fat Caesar dressing

  1 c. mixed berries

SUPPLEMENTS

  • 2 ABC Cooling Vitamin Mixture with breakfast

  • 100 mg 5-HTP one hour after dinner

  • 300 mg EPA three times a day with food

  • 200 mg DHA three times a day with food

  • 30 mg 5-HTP in sublingual pearls. Take as needed throughout the day for calming and cooling.

WEEK TWO

This week's theme is to do the best you can and be nice to yourself. Be a good friend, good parent, and/or good spouse or partner. Work hard but not too hard. Try to make the world a better place. That's all anyone can do. You're going to make mistakes—everyone does. So lighten up and give yourself permission to do so. Mistakes or setbacks, whether they're personal or professional, can be wonderful learning experiences and growth opportunities.

This week, you'll take your exercise program up a notch by adding a brisk ten-minute walk to your ten minutes of morning stretching. Continue doing twenty minutes of light, relaxing stretching in the evening. Again, do these exercises in addition to your regular workout (if you already have one).

This week we'll also make a few changes to your supplements and continue the sleep hygiene process.

Day 8

Perspective

Today's mission statement is: I love and forgive myself as I would a dear friend. I accept forgiveness from myself and others.

Sleep

Keep a sleep diary. Write down what time you got into bed, about what time you think you fell asleep, how many times you woke up in the middle of the night and how long you were awake, and what time you woke up in the morning. Don't obsess over the details, though. The last thing you need is something else to worry about.

Exercise

After you do your ten minutes of morning stretches, get dressed and take a brisk, ten-minute walk around the neighborhood. Finish your day with twenty minutes of light, relaxing stretching.

Lifestyle

Treat yourself to a glass of wine with dinner (if you're alcoholic, have a hot chocolate instead). In the evening, increase your meditation to fifteen minutes, starting at least ninety minutes before bedtime.

Diet and Supplements

You should be drinking liquid with and between meals, throughout the day. Drink half an ounce of liquid per pound of body weight (if you weigh 130 pounds, that's 65 ounces). But whatever your weight, make sure you get at least 64 ounces every day. Water (with or without lemon) and calming herbal teas such as chamomile, white, or valerian teas are fine, but caffeinated drinks, alcohol, and fruit juices don't count.

BREAKFAST

    ½ c. oatmeal with chopped almonds

    ⅓ c. cottage cheese mixed into the oatmeal or eaten separately

    1 c. fruit cocktail in juice

LUNCH

    1 toasted cheese sandwich (part skim) on whole wheat bread

    1 c. tossed mixed vegetable salad with 1½ T. low-fat dressing

    4 oz. low-fat soy or vegetable chips

    1 apple

DINNER

    Barbecue chicken:

        4 oz. chicken, white or dark meat baked with 2 T. barbecue sauce

    ½ c. baked beans

    2 pieces cornbread

    1 c. tossed green salad

    1 piece angel food cake topped with 4 oz. sliced strawberries

SUPPLEMENTS

- 3 ABC Cooling Vitamin Mixture; 2 with breakfast, 1 more with dinner
- 100 mg 5-HTP one hour after dinner
- 300 mg EPA two times a day with food
- 200 mg DHA two times a day with food
- 30 mg 5-HTP in sublingual pearls. Take as needed throughout the day for calming and cooling.

Day 9

Perspective

I can take care of myself, but I allow others to take care of me when it is appropriate.

Sleep

Stick to your weekday routine on the weekends. It's tempting to sleep in on Saturday and Sunday mornings, but doing so disrupts your biological clock and will make it even harder to get up on time feeling refreshed on Monday.

Exercise

Make a firm commitment to your ten-minute walk and promise that you'll do it rain or shine. Keep up the ten-minute morning and twenty-minute evening stretches.

Lifestyle

Sit by a body of water, whether it's a river, a stream, a lake, or the ocean. Just sit and watch the water as it moves. In the evening, increase your meditation to fifteen minutes, starting at least ninety minutes before bedtime.

Diet and Supplements

You should be drinking liquid with and between meals, throughout the day. Drink half an ounce of liquid per pound of body weight (if you weigh 130 pounds, that's 65 ounces). But whatever your weight, make sure you get at least 64 ounces every day. Water (with or without lemon) and calming herbal teas such as chamomile, white, or valerian teas are fine, but caffeinated drinks, alcohol, and fruit juices don't count.

BREAKFAST
- 1 c. Cheerios
- 1 slice whole grain toast with trans fat–free or soy margarine
- 3 slices of low-fat turkey bacon
- ½ c. low-fat milk

LUNCH
- 1 veggie dog on whole wheat bun
- 4 oz. baked potato chips
- carrot and celery sticks with 1 T. nonfat blue cheese dressing
- 1 orange

DINNER
- 4 oz. grilled salmon marinated in:
    - ½ T. wasabi
    - ¾ t. sesame oil
    - ¼ c. dry white wine
    - ¾ t. rice vinegar
- 1 c. steamed brown rice

1 c. steamed broccoli

1 c. fruit cocktail

SUPPLEMENTS

- 3 ABC Cooling Vitamin Mixture; 2 with breakfast, 1 more with dinner
- 100 mg 5-HTP one hour after dinner
- 300 mg EPA twice a day with food
- 200 mg DHA twice a day with food
- 30 mg 5-HTP in sublingual pearls. Take as needed throughout the day for calming and cooling.

Day 10

Perspective

I am lovable and I deserved to be loved even though I sometimes make mistakes.

Sleep

If you can't sleep, get out of bed. Thrashing around, looking at the clock, and getting angry that you can't fall asleep will only make it worse. While you're up, you might want to go online and find a list of the world's most boring books and make a note to check a few out of the library tomorrow.

Exercise

Continue with your ten-minute stretch, ten-minute brisk walk, and twenty-minute evening stretch. Vary your walks and the order of your stretches. Routines are great, but they can get boring after a while.

Lifestyle

Get some light. Experiments with seasonal affective disorder and exposure to the sun and/or light boxes/solar exposure indicate that light exposure raises serotonin levels. "Ott" lamps or full spectrum lighting that generates 5,000 to 10,000 lux are relatively inexpensive ($50 to $100) and can significantly increase cooling NT activity. Too much, though, can be a problem. People with bipolar disorder often have negative reactions to extremely bright conditions, and bright lights are a common migraine trigger. In the evening, increase your meditation to fifteen minutes, starting at least ninety minutes before bedtime.

Diet and Supplements

You should be drinking liquid with and between meals, throughout the day. Drink half an ounce of liquid per pound of body weight (if you weigh 130 pounds, that's 65 ounces). But whatever your weight, make sure you get at least 64 ounces every day. Water (with or without lemon) and calming herbal teas such as chamomile, white, or valerian teas are fine, but caffeinated drinks, alcohol, and fruit juices don't count.

BREAKFAST

1 c. oatmeal, with 1 scoop (16 g) soy protein powder stirred in

1 T. raw honey

1 sliced banana

1 c. low-fat milk

LUNCH

1 piece whole wheat pita bread stuffed with:

    2 oz. feta cheese

    ½ c. chickpeas

    1 c. sliced tomato and cucumber

1 T. chopped olives drizzled with 1 T. olive oil, pinch of salt

1 c. nonfat plain yogurt with 1 T. honey, 2 T. roasted, unsalted almonds

1 c. fresh sliced peaches

DINNER

4 steamed shrimp dumplings with 1 t. low sodium soy sauce

½ c. steamed edamame

1 c. steamed brown rice

1 c. tapioca pudding made with nonfat milk

SUPPLEMENTS

- 3 ABC Cooling Vitamin Mixture; 2 with breakfast, 1 more with dinner
- 100 mg 5-HTP one hour after dinner
- 300 mg EPA twice a day with food
- 200 mg DHA twice a day with food
- 30 mg 5-HTP in sublingual pearls. Take as needed throughout the day for calming and cooling.

Day 11

Perspective

I accept the people around me as they are now.

Sleep

Work out. Keep doing the exercises that are part of this plan, but not within an hour of going to bed.

Exercise

Same workout as this whole week. When taking your morning walk, be sure to swing your arms broadly. That'll get your heart pumping a little more and will increase the effectiveness of your workout.

Lifestyle

Call an old friend you haven't spoken to for a long time and catch up. In the evening, increase your meditation to fifteen minutes, starting at least ninety minutes before bedtime.

Diet and Supplements

You should be drinking liquid with and between meals, throughout the day. Drink half an ounce of liquid per pound of body weight (if you weigh 130 pounds, that's 65 ounces). But whatever your weight, make sure you get at least 64 ounces every day. Water (with or without lemon) and calming herbal teas such as chamomile, white, or valerian teas are fine, but caffeinated drinks, alcohol, and fruit juices don't count.

BREAKFAST
    1 c. cornflakes with ½ c. low-fat milk, sweetened with stevia to taste
    1 orange
    1 slice whole wheat toast with 1 t. trans fat–free margarine

LUNCH
    2 ground extra lean turkey (¼ lb.)
    soft tacos with:
        ½ sliced tomato
        2 oz. part-skim shredded cheese
        1 T. olives
        shredded lettuce
        2 T. salsa on nonfat corn tortillas
    1 banana

DINNER

    1 skinless chicken breast, grilled

    1 baked potato with 2 T. nonfat sour cream, sliced green onions

    1 c. steamed asparagus

    ½ c. nonfat frozen yogurt

SUPPLEMENTS

- 3 ABC Cooling Vitamin Mixture; 2 with breakfast, 1 more with dinner
- 100 mg 5-HTP one hour after dinner
- 300 mg EPA twice a day with food
- 200 mg DHA twice a day with food
- 30 mg 5-HTP in sublingual pearls. Take as needed throughout the day for calming and cooling.

Day 12

Perspective

I appreciate the uniqueness of the contributions I make to the world.

Sleep

Get some sun during the day. Sunlight stimulates serotonin production, which reduces your cooling deficit.

Exercise

Besides your ten-minute morning walk, your goal is to do a total of thirty minutes of stretching or light exercise every day—ten minutes in the morning and twenty more in the evening. However, the *when* isn't as important as the *how much*. Take frequent breaks at work and do a little stretching at your desk. You can even get screen savers that will remind you.

Lifestyle

Go to a bookstore or the library and find a copy of your favorite childhood book. Take it home and read it to yourself. In the evening, increase your meditation to fifteen minutes, starting at least ninety minutes before bedtime.

Diet and Supplements

You should be drinking liquid with and between meals, throughout the day. Drink half an ounce of liquid per pound of body weight (if you weigh 130 pounds, that's 65 ounces). But whatever your weight, make sure you get at least 64 ounces every day. Water (with or without lemon) and calming herbal teas such as chamomile, white, or valerian teas are fine, but caffeinated drinks, alcohol, and fruit juices don't count.

BREAKFAST

 2 whole wheat pancakes topped with ½ c. sliced strawberries or 2 T. fruit preserves

 1 c. low-fat milk

LUNCH

 6 oz. chili with vegetables or meat

 4 fat-free crackers

 green salad with tomatoes, cucumbers, celery, and 1 T. nonfat dressing

 ½ c. seedless grapes

DINNER

 Pasta salad:

   2 c. pasta of choice
   ¼ c. steamed spinach
   ¼ c. steamed carrots
   ¼ c. steamed mushrooms
   2 fresh tomato slices
   1 T. nonfat Caesar dressing

 1 c. Tofutti nondairy ice cream

SUPPLEMENTS

- 3 ABC Cooling Vitamin Mixture; 2 with breakfast, 1 more with dinner
- 100 mg 5-HTP one hour after dinner
- 300 mg EPA twice a day with food
- 200 mg DHA twice a day with food
- 30 mg 5-HTP in sublingual pearls. Take as needed throughout the day for calming and cooling.

Day 13

Perspective

I accept validation and praise for the things I do.

Sleep

Slow down before bed. Take a warm bath, have some cocoa, read quietly. Also avoid wrestling with the kids, or anything else that might rev you up, for at least an hour before sleep.

Exercise

Continue this week's workout. Be patient with yourself. It took some time to get out of shape and it'll take some time to get back in.

Lifestyle

Participate in a religious service, preferably a calm, contemplative one. In the evening, increase your meditation to fifteen minutes, starting at least ninety minutes before bedtime.

Diet and Supplements

You should be drinking liquid with and between meals, throughout the day. Drink half an ounce of liquid per pound of body weight (if you weigh 130 pounds, that's 65 ounces). But whatever your weight, make sure you get at least 64 ounces every day. Water (with or without lemon) and calming herbal teas such as chamomile, white, or valerian teas are fine, but caffeinated drinks, alcohol, and fruit juices don't count.

BREAKFAST

> 4 egg whites, scrambled
>
> 2 slices whole grain toast
>
> 1 c. fresh berries
>
> 1 T. Smart Balance spread

LUNCH

> Chicken breast sandwich:
>> 3 oz. smoked chicken breast
>>
>> 2 slices whole grain bread
>>
>> 1 T. low-fat mayonnaise
>>
>> lettuce and tomato

Green salad with cucumber and orange slices, carrots, almonds

1 T. low-fat dressing

1 kiwi

DINNER

4 oz. grilled scrod fish

1 c. steamed vegetables and garlic

Mashed potatoes topped with cashews

6 oz. low-fat yogurt with fruit

SUPPLEMENTS

- 3 ABC Cooling Vitamin Mixture; 2 with breakfast, 1 more with dinner
- 100 mg 5-HTP one hour after dinner
- 300 mg EPA twice a day with food
- 200 mg DHA twice a day with food
- 30 mg 5-HTP in sublingual pearls. Take as needed throughout the day for calming and cooling.

Day 14

Perspective

I am better able to love myself and others when I am rested and relaxed.

Sleep

Institute a bedtime routine—a pattern of activities that tells your body it's time to sleep. Brush your teeth, floss, lay out your clothes for the next day, set the alarm clock, turn out the lights. Whatever the routine, do it the same way every night.

Exercise

Same workout. The only difference today is that when you're finished, do something to reward yourself. Go out to a movie or play, hang out with some friends, or have a dessert or other food treat that you enjoy (we won't tell).

Lifestyle

Visit a museum and spend ten or fifteen minutes admiring something you find beautiful. In the evening, increase your meditation to fifteen minutes, starting at least ninety minutes before bedtime.

Diet and Supplements

You should be drinking liquid with and between meals, throughout the day. Drink half an ounce of liquid per pound of body weight (if you weigh 130 pounds, that's 65 ounces). But whatever your weight, make sure you get at least 64 ounces every day. Water (with or without lemon) and calming herbal teas such as chamomile, white, or valerian teas are fine, but caffeinated drinks, alcohol, and fruit juices don't count.

BREAKFAST

    Ham and cheese melt (cooked in oven or microwave):
- 1 slice whole wheat bread
- 2 slices low-fat ham
- 2 slices low-fat cheese of your choice

    1 apple

LUNCH

- 3 oz. sliced roast beef
- 2 slices whole wheat bread
- 2 slices tomato
- iceberg lettuce to taste
- 1 T. mustard or low-fat mayonnaise
- salt and pepper to taste
- Unlimited carrot and celery sticks

DINNER

    Veggie burger:
- 1 veggie burger patty
- 2 slices whole grain bread
- lettuce, tomato slices, onion slices
- 1 T. low-fat mayonnaise

    1 orange, sliced

    1 c. lemon sorbet with blueberries

SUPPLEMENTS

- 3 ABC Cooling Vitamin Mixture; 2 with breakfast, 1 more with dinner
- 100 mg 5-HTP one hour after dinner
- 300 mg EPA twice a day with food
- 200 mg DHA twice a day with food
- 30 mg 5-HTP in sublingual pearls. Take as needed throughout the day for calming and cooling.

WEEK THREE

This week's theme is to reward yourself. Keep a list of your goals, your thoughts, and your actions. When you do something well or accomplish a goal—even if it's a small one—do something to celebrate. And remember to do fun things, things that make you laugh.

Now that the sleep hygiene process is complete, you should be enjoying more refreshing sleep. This week we want to add some basic relaxation techniques that will further improve your sleeping experience. The simplest approach is to simply concentrate on your breath. Feel the air coming into your lungs and imagine it spreading throughout your body, all the way to the tips of your fingers and toes. Hold the breath for a few seconds and slowly exhale, imagining the breath leaving your body and disappearing into the air around you. If you feel tension in a particular body part, make a conscious effort to relax whatever it is that's tense. Think only of your breath. If you find your mind wandering, bring your thoughts back to your breath.

Another effective technique is guided imagery. Start off by doing some deep breathing until you feel relaxed. Then imagine yourself walking in the most peaceful, quiet place you've ever been, all alone. Keep walking, admiring the scenery, the plants, the smell of the air.

This week you'll take your exercise routine up another notch. Replace your morning walk and stretching routine with twenty minutes of intense aerobic exercise. Continue doing twenty minutes of stretching in the evening but vary your routine. If you're already doing another fitness program, eliminate one workout a week.

Day 15

Perspective

Today's mission statement is: I have the right to be treated with respect by those around me and the courage to stand up for myself when I'm not getting what I need.

Sleep

Keep up your sleep hygiene routine. Add in fifteen to twenty minutes of deep relaxation or guided imagery.

Exercise

Twenty minutes of intense aerobic exercise in the morning and twenty minutes of relaxing stretching in the evening. For the aerobic part of the workout, find an activity that you enjoy and that you think you'll realistically be able to stick with for at least a few weeks.

Lifestyle

Try acupuncture. Acupuncture has been shown to be effective in relieving pain, reducing inflammation, and treating obesity—all of which are conditions that are related to increasing serotonin levels. In addition, increase your meditation time to fifteen minutes twice a day. That may be hard, given your tendency to overbook your time. If you can't do fifteen minutes twice a day, try for twenty minutes once. Regardless of how much time you commit to meditating, be sure to schedule your sessions for times when you're not in a rush.

Diet and Supplements

You should be drinking liquid with and between meals, throughout the day. Drink half an ounce of liquid per pound of body weight (if you weigh 130 pounds, that's 65 ounces). But whatever your weight, make sure you get at least 64 ounces every day. Water (with or without lemon) and calming herbal teas such as chamomile, white, or valerian teas are fine, but caffeinated drinks, alcohol, and fruit juices don't count.

BREAKFAST

    1 c. low-fat cottage cheese

    ½ c. peaches in juice

2 slices raisin toast

1 T. Smart Balance spread

LUNCH

Turkey salad (mixed and served on Bibb lettuce):

> 4 oz. chopped turkey
>
> 1 T. low-fat mayonnaise
>
> 12 raisins or 12 sliced grapes
>
> 1 diced apple
>
> ¼ c. chopped walnuts

2 whole grain breadsticks

DINNER

4 oz. barbecued chicken

1 c. steamed green beans

½ c. Rice-a-Roni

green salad with tomato slices, cucumber

1 T. olive oil and 1 T. fresh lemon juice

1 nonfat fudgesicle

SUPPLEMENTS

- 3 ABC Cooling Vitamin Mixture; 2 with breakfast, 1 more with dinner
- 100 mg 5-HTP one hour after dinner
- 300 mg EPA twice a day with food
- 200 mg DHA twice a day with food
- 30 mg 5-HTP in sublingual pearls. Take as needed throughout the day for calming and cooling.

Day 16

Perspective

Today I will do something based on my intuition and I will resist the temptation to second-guess myself.

Sleep

Keep up your sleep hygiene routine. Add in fifteen to twenty minutes of deep relaxation or guided imagery.

Exercise

Same workout as yesterday: twenty minutes of aerobic exercise in the morning and twenty minutes of relaxing stretching in the evening.

Lifestyle

Create a silent zone in your home, a place you can go for thirty minutes without being interrupted by the phone, e-mail, the doorbell, or requests for homework help. This is in addition to the meditation, which you're doing fifteen minutes twice a day or twenty minutes once a day.

Diet and Supplements

You should be drinking liquid with and between meals, throughout the day. Drink half an ounce of liquid per pound of body weight (if you weigh 130 pounds, that's 65 ounces). But whatever your weight, make sure you get at least 64 ounces every day. Water (with or without lemon) and calming herbal teas such as chamomile, white, or valerian teas are fine, but caffeinated drinks, alcohol, and fruit juices don't count.

BREAKFAST

 1 c. cold cereal

 1 c. low-fat milk

 1 c. fresh berries

 1 slice whole grain toast with trans fat–free margarine

LUNCH

 1 c. minestrone soup

 4 oz. poached salmon

 1 c. steamed broccoli and summer squash

 1 dinner roll

DINNER

 8 oz. scrambled tofu with:

  ½ c. broccoli

  garlic

  soy sauce

  2 T. olive oil

 1½ c. brown rice

1 c. tossed green salad with 1 T. low-fat dressing

1 apple

SUPPLEMENTS

- 3 ABC Cooling Vitamin Mixture; 2 with breakfast, 1 more with dinner
- 100 mg 5-HTP one hour after dinner
- 300 mg EPA twice a day with food
- 200 mg DHA twice a day with food
- 30 mg 5-HTP in sublingual pearls. Take as needed throughout the day for calming and cooling.

Day 17

Perspective

There is far more to me than my job, my income, or where I live.

Sleep

Keep up your sleep hygiene routine. Add in fifteen to twenty minutes of deep relaxation or guided imagery.

Exercise

Twenty minutes of aerobic exercise in the morning and twenty minutes of relaxing stretching in the evening. If you're feeling frustrated with your progress and need a little motivation, work out with a partner— preferably someone who's in slightly better shape than you and can give you the encouragement you need.

Lifestyle

Give someone you love an extra-long hug. Being touched, hugged, caressed, and held all stimulate serotonin release, which makes you feel safe and loved. Increase your meditation time to fifteen minutes twice a day or twenty minutes once.

Diet and Supplements

You should be drinking liquid with and between meals, throughout the day. Drink half an ounce of liquid per pound of body weight (if you weigh 130 pounds, that's 65 ounces). But whatever your weight, make sure you get at least 64 ounces every day. Water (with or without lemon) and calming herbal teas such as chamomile, white, or valerian teas are fine, but caffeinated drinks, alcohol, and fruit juices don't count.

BREAKFAST

½ c. Grape Nuts cereal

½ sliced banana

1 c. low-fat milk

1 English muffin with 1 T. fruit preserves

LUNCH

5 oz. tuna (water-pack)

2 T. low-fat dressing

1 c. diced carrots and celery

2 slices whole grain toast

1 c. tossed salad with 1 T. dressing

1 orange

DINNER

1 c. brown rice, cooked, stir fried with:

>   1 c. steamed vegetables
>   2 scrambled eggs
>   1 clove garlic, minced
>   1 t. olive oil

1 slice pineapple

1 c. mixed berries

SUPPLEMENTS

- 3 ABC Cooling Vitamin Mixture; 2 with breakfast, 1 more with dinner
- 100 mg 5-HTP one hour after dinner
- 300 mg EPA twice a day with food
- 200 mg DHA twice a day with food
- 30 mg 5-HTP in sublingual pearls. Take as needed throughout the day for calming and cooling.

Day 18

Perspective

Today I will find something good in my life to be grateful for and I will practice thoughts of gratitude.

Sleep

Keep up your sleep hygiene routine. Add in fifteen to twenty minutes of deep relaxation or guided imagery.

Exercise

Same workout as the rest of this week: twenty minutes of aerobic exercise in the morning and twenty minutes of relaxing stretching in the evening.

Lifestyle

Have an electricity-free day—no computer, no phone, no pager, no television, no car. Rediscover all the wonderful things there are to do without using power. Include meditation time fifteen minutes twice a day or twenty minutes once a day.

Diet and Supplements

You should be drinking liquid with and between meals, throughout the day. Drink half an ounce of liquid per pound of body weight (if you weigh 130 pounds, that's 65 ounces). But whatever your weight, make sure you get at least 64 ounces every day. Water (with or without lemon) and calming herbal teas such as chamomile, white, or valerian teas are fine, but caffeinated drinks, alcohol, and fruit juices don't count.

BREAKFAST

    2 slices French toast made with 3 eggs

    1 T. fruit preserves

    4 oz. nonfat plain yogurt

LUNCH

    1 toasted cheese sandwich (part-skim) on whole wheat bread

    1 c. tossed mixed vegetable salad with 1½ T. low-fat dressing

    4 oz. soy chips

    1 pear

Dinner

    4 oz. grilled salmon

    1 c. sliced tomatoes with 1 T. olive oil, salt, garlic powder, lemon

    2 T. low-fat dressing

    2 c. steamed quinoa

    1 c. squash sautéed in olive oil

    1 c. mixed berries

Supplements

- 3 ABC Cooling Vitamin Mixture; 2 with breakfast, 1 more with dinner
- 100 mg 5-HTP one hour after dinner
- 300 mg EPA twice a day with food
- 200 mg DHA twice a day with food
- 30 mg 5-HTP in sublingual pearls. Take as needed throughout the day for calming and cooling.

Day 19

Perspective

Today I will forgive someone and I will seek the forgiveness of another.

Sleep

Keep up your sleep hygiene routine. Add in fifteen to twenty minutes of deep relaxation or guided imagery.

Exercise

Twenty minutes of aerobic exercise in the morning and twenty minutes of relaxing stretching in the evening. Calculate your target heart rate for working out (60 percent to 80 percent of the number that's 220 minus your age). Take your pulse a few times during the aerobic part of your workout to make sure you're in the zone.

Lifestyle

Play with a puppy at the local animal shelter. Maintain your meditation time at fifteen minutes twice a day or twenty minutes once a day.

Diet and Supplements

You should be drinking liquid with and between meals, throughout the day. Drink half an ounce of liquid per pound of body weight (if you weigh 130 pounds, that's 65 ounces). But whatever your weight, make sure you get at least 64 ounces every day. Water (with or without lemon) and calming herbal teas such as chamomile, white, or valerian teas are fine, but caffeinated drinks, alcohol, and fruit juices don't count.

BREAKFAST

    8 oz. low-fat yogurt with fruit

    ½ scoop (8 g) whey protein powder with 2 T. chopped nuts of your choice mixed in

LUNCH

    5 oz. chicken breast

    2 slices whole grain toast

    2 T. low-fat mayonnaise

    1 sliced tomato

    1 carrot

    1 apple

DINNER

    4 oz. grilled fresh cod marinated with:

        ½ T. wasabi

        ¾ t. sesame oil

        ¼ c. dry white wine

        ¾ t. rice vinegar

    1 c. cooked couscous

    1 c. spinach sautéed in olive oil with fresh chopped garlic

    1 c. fruit cocktail

SUPPLEMENTS

- 3 ABC Cooling Vitamin Mixture; 2 with breakfast, 1 more with dinner
- 100 mg 5-HTP one hour after dinner
- 300 mg EPA twice a day with food
- 200 mg DHA twice a day with food
- 30 mg 5-HTP in sublingual pearls. Take as needed throughout the day for calming and cooling.

Day 20

Perspective

I am important to myself and to others. I will make time to relax, rest, and care for myself.

Sleep

Keep up your sleep hygiene routine. Add in fifteen to twenty minutes of deep relaxation or guided imagery.

Exercise

Twenty minutes of aerobic exercise in the morning and twenty minutes of relaxing stretching in the evening. If you're working out with a tape or a television show, try to follow the routine that makes you work. If you're not sweating after twenty minutes, you're not working hard enough.

Lifestyle

Listen to slow, melodic music—no rock, no rap, no heavy metal. Maintain your meditation time at fifteen minutes twice a day or twenty minutes once a day.

Diet and Supplements

You should be drinking liquid with and between meals, throughout the day. Drink half an ounce of liquid per pound of body weight (if you weigh 130 pounds, that's 65 ounces). But whatever your weight, make sure you get at least 64 ounces every day. Water (with or without lemon) and calming herbal teas such as chamomile, white, or valerian teas are fine, but caffeinated drinks, alcohol, and fruit juices don't count.

BREAKFAST

    1½ c. cornflakes

    1 c. nonfat milk

    ½ c. sliced peaches in juice

    2 pieces Canadian bacon

LUNCH

    Turkey burger:

        4 oz. grilled low-fat turkey meat

> 1 whole wheat bun
> 1 T. ketchup
> slices iceberg lettuce

4 oz. low-fat soy or vegetable chips

carrot and celery sticks with 1 T. nonfat ranch dressing

DINNER

5 oz. beef tenderloin cooked to taste

8 steamed asparagus spears

1 c. brown rice

1 c. tossed green salad with 1 T. lemon juice and 1 T. olive oil

1 c. cubed honeydew melon

SUPPLEMENTS

- 3 ABC Cooling Vitamin Mixture; 2 with breakfast, 1 more with dinner
- 100 mg 5-HTP one hour after dinner
- 300 mg EPA twice a day with food
- 200 mg DHA twice a day with food
- 30 mg 5-HTP in sublingual pearls. Take as needed throughout the day for calming and cooling.

Day 21

Perspective

I am thankful for the valuable lessons I've learned from life.

Sleep

Keep up your sleep hygiene routine. Add in fifteen to twenty minutes of deep relaxation or guided imagery.

Exercise

Twenty minutes of aerobic exercise in the morning and twenty minutes of relaxing stretching in the evening. Get a tape or CD and listen to some music or a book on tape while you're working out.

Lifestyle

Take an extra-long lunch and sign up for a yoga class. Maintain your meditation time at fifteen minutes twice a day or twenty minutes once a day.

Diet and Supplements

You should be drinking liquid with and between meals, throughout the day. Drink half an ounce of liquid per pound of body weight (if you weigh 130 pounds, that's 65 ounces). But whatever your weight, make sure you get at least 64 ounces every day. Water (with or without lemon) and calming herbal teas such as chamomile, white, or valerian teas are fine, but caffeinated drinks, alcohol, and fruit juices don't count.

BREAKFAST

1 c. slow-cooked oatmeal with 1 T. nuts, sweetened to taste with cinnamon and stevia or ½ T. raw honey

¾ c. berries

4 slices pan-grilled turkey

LUNCH

4-egg-white omelet with 3 oz. low-fat cheese

1 c. steamed vegetables

½ c. salsa

2 whole grain breadsticks

DINNER

Chicken Caesar salad:

    4 oz. grilled chicken, cubed

    1 c. romaine lettuce

    1 T. low-fat Caesar dressing

    1 t. grated low-fat parmesan cheese

    ¼ c. seasoned whole wheat croutons

2 figs or 1 c. diced apple mixed with cinnamon and 20 golden raisins

SUPPLEMENTS

- 3 ABC Cooling Vitamin Mixture; 2 with breakfast, 1 more with dinner
- 100 mg 5-HTP one hour after dinner
- 300 mg EPA twice a day with food
- 200 mg DHA twice a day with food
- 30 mg 5-HTP in sublingual pearls. Take as needed throughout the day for calming and cooling.

WEEK FOUR

Congratulations, you're almost there. This week's theme is to keep your eyes open. Sometimes, no matter what you do, life isn't going to be as rosy as you'd like. When that happens, carefully evaluate the situation. What will you do if the worst happens? Be honest.

This week we'll make a few more small adjustments to your supplements and your exercise program. If you're still having trouble sleeping, we have one more approach that we want you to try. It's called *progressive muscle relaxation* (PMR) and it works like this:

Start by doing a few minutes of deep breathing, until you feel relatively relaxed. Then focus your thoughts on a particular group of muscles—your arms, for example. Tighten the muscles and keep them tight until you start to feel some pain. Then relax and notice how wonderful it feels when the blood floods back into the tissue. After twenty seconds of relaxing, do it again. Then do the same thing on the other side. You'll start the week off doing this exercise with your arms. Over the next few days you'll add in your legs, back, stomach, and neck, and by the end of the week you'll be doing your whole body.

This week you'll vary your workouts and increase your exercise time even more. You'll be doing some kind of resistance or weight training three times a week and at least twenty to thirty minutes of aerobic exercise on the non–weight training days. Continue doing twenty minutes of gentle, relaxing stretching in the evening—it'll feel great.

Day 22

Perspective

Today's mission statement is: I will concentrate on making progress, not on achieving perfection.

Sleep

Do PMR, starting with your right side. Tense and relax your fist as described above. After you've done this twice, do the same thing with your left fist.

Exercise

Today's a resistance training day. If you have weights or are a member of a club that has weights, use them. But take it easy for this first workout: work each area of your body using about 50 to 60 percent of the weight you think you can handle. If you're an experienced exerciser, go ahead and do your regular weight training routine. Round out your day with twenty minutes of gentle, relaxing stretching in the evening.

Lifestyle

Get a massage. An experienced massage therapist will perform techniques that stimulate the increase of both warming and cooling NTs, but in a way that allows your nervous system to choose the dominant neurotransmitter. A recent study published in the *Journal of Clinical Rheumatology* found that massage therapy helped fibromyalgia patients sleep more and decreased their sleep movements. Continue doing fifteen minutes of meditation twice a day or twenty minutes once a day.

Diet and Supplements

You should be drinking liquid with and between meals, throughout the day. Drink half an ounce of liquid per pound of body weight (if you weigh 130 pounds, that's 65 ounces). But whatever your weight, make sure you get at least 64 ounces every day. Water (with or without lemon) and calming herbal teas such as chamomile, white, or valerian teas are fine, but caffeinated drinks, alcohol, and fruit juices don't count.

BREAKFAST

    2 cheese blintzes

    1 T. pineapple or apple preserves

    1 c. skim milk

LUNCH

    1 piece whole wheat pita bread stuffed with:

        2 oz. feta cheese

        ½ c. chickpeas

        1 c. sliced tomato and cucumber

        1 T. chopped olives drizzled with 1 T. olive oil

        pinch of salt

    1 c. nonfat plain yogurt with 1 T. honey, 2 T. roasted, unsalted filberts

    1 tangerine

DINNER

    1½ c. yankee bean soup

    4 oz. grilled sirloin (lean)

2 c. chickpea salad with chopped tomato, red pepper, garlic and balsamic dressing

1 c. tossed salad with 2 T. low-fat dressing

1 glass red wine

sliced strawberries

Supplements

- 3 ABC Cooling Vitamin Mixture; 2 with breakfast, 2 more with dinner
- 100 mg 5-HTP one hour after dinner
- 300 mg EPA twice a day with food
- 200 mg DHA twice a day with food
- 30 mg 5-HTP in sublingual pearls. Take as needed throughout the day for calming and cooling.

Day 23

Perspective

I will remember that isolation serves no purpose in my life.

Sleep

PMR. Start with your right fist, as described yesterday. Then continue with your bicep. After you've done the right arm twice, do the same thing with your left.

Exercise

Twenty to thirty minutes of aerobics this morning and twenty minutes of gentle, relaxing stretching in the evening. Join a class at your local Y or health club and do a step aerobics or intensive aerobics class.

Lifestyle

Write a love letter. Getting in touch with deep emotions helps release serotonin. Continue doing fifteen minutes of meditation twice a day or twenty minutes once a day.

Diet and Supplements

You should be drinking liquid with and between meals, throughout the day. Drink half an ounce of liquid per pound of body weight (if you weigh 130 pounds, that's 65 ounces). But whatever your weight, make sure you get at least 64 ounces every day. Water (with or without lemon) and calming herbal teas such as chamomile, white, or valerian teas are fine, but caffeinated drinks, alcohol, and fruit juices don't count.

BREAKFAST

1½ c. of puffed rice or millet cereal sweetened with stevia or Splenda to taste

1 c. nonfat milk

1 banana

2 low-fat turkey sausages

LUNCH

2 c. lentil salad with:

½ c. diced tomato and celery

1 c. corn with 2 t. dressing

2 whole grain breadsticks

1 c. tossed green salad

1 T. low-fat dressing

DINNER

1 skinless chicken breast, grilled

1 baked potato with 2 T. nonfat sour cream, sliced green onions

1 c. peas

½ c. mixed berries

1 glass red wine

SUPPLEMENTS

- 3 ABC Cooling Vitamin Mixture; 2 with breakfast, 1 more with dinner
- 100 mg 5-HTP one hour after dinner
- 300 mg EPA twice a day with food
- 200 mg DHA twice a day with food
- 30 mg 5-HTP in sublingual pearls. Take as needed throughout the day for calming and cooling.

Day 24

Perspective

Asking for help when I need it is a sign of strength, not weakness.

Sleep

PMR. Do both arms. Then add your right foot, tensing your toes tightly until they hurt, and then relaxing. After you do your toes, do your calf. When you've finished your right foot and calf, do the left.

Exercise

Resistance training today with twenty minutes of gentle, relaxing stretching in the evening. When doing your weights, concentrate on good form: lift with your legs, not your back; don't hunch over; don't overdo the weight; and avoid jerky, sudden movements.

Lifestyle

Treat yourself to a facial, manicure, and pedicure—even if you're a man. Continue doing fifteen minutes of meditation twice a day or twenty minutes once a day.

Diet and Supplements

You should be drinking liquid with and between meals, throughout the day. Drink half an ounce of liquid per pound of body weight (if you weigh 130 pounds, that's 65 ounces). But whatever your weight, make sure you get at least 64 ounces every day. Water (with or without lemon) and calming herbal teas such as chamomile, white, or valerian teas are fine, but caffeinated drinks, alcohol, and fruit juices don't count.

BREAKFAST

    2 whole grain buckwheat pancakes

    1 c. low-fat yogurt

    1 apple

LUNCH

    2 ground extra lean turkey (¼ lb.)

    soft tacos with:

        ½ sliced tomato

        2 oz. part-skim shredded cheese

        1 T. olives

        shredded lettuce

        2 T. salsa on nonfat corn tortillas

    ½ c. grapes

DINNER

- 6 oz. grilled orange roughy
- 1 c. wild rice
- 1 c. tossed green salad with 2 T. low-fat dressing
- 1 whole grain dinner roll
- 1 glass white wine
- 1 pear

SUPPLEMENTS

- 3 ABC Cooling Vitamin Mixture; 2 with breakfast, 1 more with dinner
- 100 mg 5-HTP one hour after dinner
- 300 mg EPA twice a day with food
- 200 mg DHA twice a day with food
- 30 mg 5-HTP in sublingual pearls. Take as needed throughout the day for calming and cooling.

Day 25

Perspective

I am aware of my limits and can say no without feeling guilty.

Sleep

PMR. Do both arms and both feet, but after you've finished with the calf, continue with the thigh and buttock. Do both sides.

Exercise

Aerobics today. Join a league and do your aerobics workout as part of a team. Don't forget your twenty-minute evening stretch.

Lifestyle

Read some favorite poetry in front of a crackling fire if possible. Continue doing fifteen minutes of meditation twice a day or twenty minutes once a day.

Diet and Supplements

You should be drinking liquid with and between meals, throughout the day. Drink half an ounce of liquid per pound of body weight (if you weigh 130 pounds, that's 65 ounces). But whatever your weight, make sure you get at least 64 ounces every day. Water (with or without lemon) and calming herbal teas such as chamomile, white, or valerian teas are fine, but caffeinated drinks, alcohol, and fruit juices don't count.

BREAKFAST

    1 c. slow-cooked oatmeal

    ½ c. skim milk

    1 T. raw honey

    1 banana

LUNCH

    3 oz. jack cheese melted between 2 slices whole grain bread

    1 c. tossed salad with 1 c. chickpeas

    1½ T. low-fat dressing

    1 kiwi

DINNER

    Chicken-beef-veggie stew:

        Brown 3 oz. raw cubed chicken and 2 oz. cubed lean beef in 1 T. olive oil

        Add ½ c. broccoli florets, ½ c. cauliflower, ¼ c. sliced celery, ¼ c. sliced carrot, ¼ c. sliced mushroom and sauté until barely soft

        Cover to simmer until cooked

        Add ½ tomato and cook, uncovered, 1 minute longer

        Season with salt and pepper to taste

    1 c. brown rice

SUPPLEMENTS

- 3 ABC Cooling Vitamin Mixture; 2 with breakfast, 1 more with dinner
- 100 mg 5-HTP one hour after dinner
- 300 mg EPA twice a day with food
- 200 mg DHA twice a day with food
- 30 mg 5-HTP in sublingual pearls. Take as needed throughout the day for calming and cooling.

Day 26

Perspective

I trust those around me to live their lives and take responsibility for their own actions. I am not responsible for what others do.

Sleep

PMR. Do both arms, this time adding in the shoulders, one at a time. Then do your legs. After that, tense and relax your stomach muscles in the same way.

Exercise

Resistance training today. Try to increase the weight you were using by 5 percent but do the same number of repetitions. Your evening stretching routine stays the same.

Lifestyle

Go for a slow walk in the woods or some other quiet place where you can be alone. Continue doing fifteen minutes of meditation twice a day or twenty minutes once a day.

Diet and Supplements

You should be drinking liquid with and between meals, throughout the day. Drink half an ounce of liquid per pound of body weight (if you weigh 130 pounds, that's 65 ounces). But whatever your weight, make sure you get at least 64 ounces every day. Water (with or without lemon) and calming herbal teas such as chamomile, white, or valerian teas are fine, but caffeinated drinks, alcohol, and fruit juices don't count.

BREAKFAST

    ½ c. Grape Nuts cereal

    1 sliced banana

    1 c. low-fat milk

    1 English muffin with 1 T. fruit preserves

LUNCH

    Pasta salad:

        2 c. pasta of choice

        ¼ c. steamed broccoli

¼ c. steamed peas

¼ c. steamed mushrooms

2 fresh tomato slices

1 T. nonfat Caesar dressing

1 c. fresh fruit cocktail

DINNER

5 oz. pan-seared sliced fresh turkey breast

2 8-in. whole wheat tortillas

1 c. shredded lettuce

1 c. chopped fresh tomato

½ c. shredded low-fat jack cheese

3 T. salsa

½ cantaloupe

SUPPLEMENTS

- 3 ABC Cooling Vitamin Mixture; 2 with breakfast, 1 more with dinner
- 100 mg 5-HTP one hour after dinner
- 300 mg EPA twice a day with food
- 200 mg DHA twice a day with food
- 30 mg 5-HTP in sublingual pearls. Take as needed throughout the day for calming and cooling.

Day 27

Perspective

I will avoid feeling guilty for things that are beyond my control.

Sleep

PMR. Do your arms, shoulders, legs, and stomach. Then add in your neck, repeating twice. After that do each eye, and finally your mouth, tightly clenching your lips.

Exercise

Do some aerobic cross-training today. If you've been running, take a bike ride or go for a swim. If you've been taking an aerobics class or using an elliptical trainer, play basketball for a while. It doesn't matter what you do, as long as it's something different from what you usually do and it makes you sweat. Keep your twenty-minute stretching routine the same, though.

Lifestyle

Spend twenty to thirty minutes writing in a journal. Continue doing fifteen minutes of meditation twice a day or twenty minutes once a day.

Diet and Supplements

You should be drinking liquid with and between meals, throughout the day. Drink half an ounce of liquid per pound of body weight (if you weigh 130 pounds, that's 65 ounces). But whatever your weight, make sure you get at least 64 ounces every day. Water (with or without lemon) and calming herbal teas such as chamomile, white, or valerian teas are fine, but caffeinated drinks, alcohol, and fruit juices don't count.

BREAKFAST

- 1 c. oatmeal, with 1 scoop (16 g) soy protein powder mixed in, with cinnamon and/or stevia to taste
- 1 sliced banana
- 1 c. low-fat milk
- 12 raisins

LUNCH

- 1 Boca burger
- 1 whole wheat bun
- 1 c. brown rice
- 1½ c. sliced tomatoes with 1 T. olive oil, salt, garlic powder, lemon
- 1 fresh nectarine

DINNER

- 4 oz. grilled salmon
- 1 c. pasta with steamed vegetables and garlic
- 1 glass red wine
- 6 oz. low-fat yogurt with fruit

SUPPLEMENTS

- 3 ABC Cooling Vitamin Mixture; 2 with breakfast, 1 more with dinner

- 100 mg 5-HTP one hour after dinner
- 300 mg EPA twice a day with food
- 200 mg DHA twice a day with food
- 30 mg 5-HTP in sublingual pearls. Take as needed throughout the day for calming and cooling.

Day 28

Perspective

I am not afraid to stand up for what I believe even if others disagree with me.

Sleep

PMR. Do your entire body. Starting with the arms, moving on to the shoulders, legs, stomach, neck, and face.

Exercise

Reward yourself with a day off! Instead of working out, spend a little time shopping for the right equipment. Be prepared to spend more than you were expecting. Good shoes in particular can make a huge difference, reducing pain, making your workouts more enjoyable, and extending the life of your knees and hips.

Lifestyle

Rent a video of a mushy love story with a happy ending. Continue doing fifteen minutes of meditation twice a day or twenty minutes once a day.

Diet and Supplements

You should be drinking liquid with and between meals, throughout the day. Drink half an ounce of liquid per pound of body weight (if you weigh 130 pounds, that's 65 ounces). But whatever your weight, make sure you get at least 64 ounces every day. Water (with or without lemon) and calming herbal teas such as chamomile, white, or valerian teas are fine, but caffeinated drinks, alcohol, and fruit juices don't count.

BREAKFAST

    4 egg whites scrambled with fresh chopped dill

    2 slices whole grain toast

    1 c. fresh sliced strawberries

    1 T. trans fat–free margarine

LUNCH

> 1 toasted low-fat American cheese sandwich on 9-grain bread
>
> 1 c. tossed mixed vegetable salad with 1½ T. low-fat dressing
>
> 4 oz. low-fat soy or vegetable chips
>
> ½ c. honeydew melon

DINNER

> 5 oz. roast lean pork tenderloin
>
> 2 c. fresh spinach sautéed in 1 T. olive oil with 2 cloves garlic, chopped
>
> 4 slices fresh pan-seared pineapple
>
> 1 glass red wine
>
> 1 c. nonfat Tofutti

SUPPLEMENTS

- 3 ABC Cooling Vitamin Mixture; 2 with breakfast, 1 more with dinner
- 100 mg 5-HTP one hour after dinner
- 300 mg EPA twice a day with food
- 200 mg DHA twice a day with food
- 30 mg 5-HTP in sublingual pearls. Take as needed throughout the day for calming and cooling.

Maintaining Your Balance

Your cooling deficiency means that you are, by nature, a little too warm for your own good, a little more active than you can afford to be, and a little more anxious than is comfortable. You might be a worrier, controlling, even obsessive at times. You might also be somewhat impulsive and quick to anger. All of these traits create their own unique challenges in your daily life, but the biggest challenge of all is that they make you vulnerable to the symptoms and diseases that are caused by true cooling deficiencies.

Maintaining your balance and staying away from deficiency isn't difficult if you consciously incorporate the following simple, cooling-stimulating lifestyle choices on a daily basis:

Prefer healthy carbohydrates.   Eat foods such as grapefruit, steel cut oats, or sprouted bread in the morning to stimulate cooling NTs that might not naturally rise in proportion to warming activity (which is strongest in the morning).

Avoid caffeine totally.   If you do consume it, postpone it until after noon and drink it between 12:00 P.M. and 6:00 P.M. for its stimulating effect, but not after that to avoid insomnia.

Eat small meals and snacks throughout the day.   The potential physical problems you face with a cooling deficiency include more inflammation than you can heal, more free radicals and oxidative stress than you can neutralize, and more energy than you can easily sustain. Eating lean protein and healthy fats such as nuts and nut butters, interspersed with snacks of healthy carbohydrates, will increase your cooling activity and minimize the detrimental effects of these potential problems.

Drink lots of water.   The ideal formula is to consume half an ounce every day for every pound of body weight. This will keep you cool and dilute the waste and damage done by the excesses of warming activity that you experience.

Upgrade your antioxidant intake.   Keep taking the cooling support supplements, vitamins E and C, omega-3 oils, EPE, DHA, and the cooling amino acid 5-HTP, in the amounts specified in the first week of this program. Add a mixed carotene supplement with minimal amounts of the most ubiquitous carotene fractions, alpha and beta carotene, and take 200 to 500 mg of alpha lipoic acid each day for extra cooling NT support.

Exercise vigorously.   Interspersing a focused workout activity such as Pilates or yoga is fine for increasing cooling NT activity. But unless you've slipped into a true cooling deficiency, exercise intensely. (If you feel that you have slipped, go back and review the exercise section of the 28-day plan.) You'll benefit from the heat created by your workout and the resulting increase in cooling NTs.

Get plenty of rest.   Sleep is particularly important to you. Your warming neurochemicals and hormones are replenished during sleep. And since you're already a little too warm, this could give you some trouble falling or staying asleep. Eat a small starchy snack such as white or sweet potato, a rice cake, or a slice of sprouted bread with raw honey or nut butter to help increase serotonin. Keep your bedroom dark to allow the full release of sleep-inducing cooling NTs. If you still have trouble sleeping, turn the lights down earlier in the evening and take a magnesium supplement to help you relax.

Schedule your exercise and shower.   Consider exercising in the afternoon and showering at night before bed. This will allow a slower,
more natural increase of warming NT activity in the morning, and
will help you sustain a steady level throughout the day. Showering in
warm or hot water will provoke higher levels of cooling NT, resulting in a natural "cool down" before bed. If you're a bath person,
adding some Epsom salts (which is actually magnesium salt) to your
bath will help relax your muscles and increase cooling activity even
more). This will help you fall asleep more easily and stay cooler and
more comfortable through the night.

Try to stay calm.   Perspective is important to the cooling-deficient disposition person every minute of every day. Your tendency is to make
too much out of things and to universalize the moment especially if
it is negative or threatening. Remind yourself that things are never as
bad as they might seem, and that the bad things you fear rarely ever
happen. You must practice letting it go and maintaining a calm and
confident perspective. Breathe deeply, stretch, smile, and take it easy.

Try to relax.   If you need help relaxing, there are a number of natural
agents that can help. The most effective is 5-HTP, which we discussed in detail in this chapter. Taking an additional 25 to 50 mg of
5-HTP sublingually (under your tongue) and an additional 100 to
200 mg orally will calm you down and keep you that way for hours.
You can carry these sublingual capsules or drops with you everywhere and use them whenever you feel overheated, anxious, restless,
or upset. You may also want to experiment with some of the other
options discussed in the 28-day plan to see whether there's anything
that might work better.

See your doctor.   If you feel yourself sliding into a serious deficiency
and need medication to keep from completely relapsing, ask your
doctor which of the cooling-enhancing drugs would be best for you.

Working with Your Doctor to Get
Back in Balance

Sometimes, despite your best efforts, you may need a little extra help
from your doctor to get your serotonin and GABA levels into the
proper balance. In these cases your physician may prescribe specialized

herbs, hormones, prescription drugs, and even biofeedback. In the following sections we'll talk about how each of these options works and what the potential side effects are. Remember, though, *do not* try any of this except as directed by your physician. Not following his or her directions or making adjustments on your own can be dangerous, if not life-threatening. For those reasons we're not including information on specific dosages. If you're interested in any of the approaches we discuss in this section, consider taking this book along next time you see your doctor.

Hormones

Hormones are natural chemicals produced by the human body. They're responsible for regulating a number of critical organ functions, are involved in cell development and repair, and help modulate our behavior. You can get many hormone precursors (the chemicals that turn into hormones after the brain and body break them down a little) without a prescription, but we strongly recommend that you consult with your physician or trained health care provider before taking any of them.

Many psychiatrists are starting to pay attention to the role of hormones in mood and memory disorders including depression, anxiety, and dementia. No hormone deficiencies have been linked to deficiencies of cooling neurotransmitters, with the possible exception of *allopregnenanole,* a neuroactive steroid that has been studied as an antianxiety drug because of its ability to stimulate GABA receptors.

Other than that, the only hormone-related way of increasing serotonin levels is to lower levels of a hormone called *corticotropin-releasing hormone* (CRH). CRH is released by the hypothalamus and directs the body's response to stress, speeding up activity in our brain, hormonal, and immune cells, gearing them up for confrontation. Several new drugs, called *CRH blockers,* are being developed, and have been shown in early trials to reduce anxiety and depression in humans and animals.

Estrogen and Hormone Replacement Therapy

One of estrogen's many functions is to improve the activity of cooling neurotransmitters in women's bodies. As estrogen production drops with age, those neurotransmitters lose some of their support. This results in many of the symptoms commonly associated with menopause.

It used to be that any menopausal woman who walked into her doctor's office complaining of hot flashes was put on estrogen for the next thirty years, no questions asked. We believe that was a mistake—one that resulted in the recent talk about how the risks of estrogen therapy may outweigh the rewards. Several of the major pharmaceutical companies have essentially pulled their estrogen drugs off the market in response to the controversy.

Simply put, for the right woman, there's nothing better than estrogen replacement. But only for the right woman. Determining who's a good candidate and who's not is done by taking a detailed family history and by ordering tests to determine hormone levels. As estrogen is metabolized, it breaks down into two products: *2 hydroxy estrone,* which is benign, and *16 hydroxy estrone,* which has been strongly implicated in the development of breast cancer. As you might expect, the ratio between the two is very important. And what tilts it one way or the other is a function of the woman's diet and lifestyle. Women who exercise and eat plenty of cruciferous vegetables (cabbage, broccoli, brussels sprouts, and cauliflower) have far lower levels of 16 hydroxy estrone and far higher levels of 2 hydroxy estrone.

After the first month on estrogen replacement, the 2:16 ratio should be rechecked. If 16s are too high the patient has to hit the gym a little harder and eat more cruciferous vegetables. (Alternatively, she could take the active cruciferous extracts *di-indole methane* and *3 indole carbinol,* both of which are widely available in supplement form.) If after another month she's unable to make the change, it's best to take her off the estrogen. In addition, women who have had (or have a family history of) breast cancer, uterine cancer, or fibrocystic breast disease need very careful evaluation by the doctor. Many of these women should not be taking estrogen, but for others it may be fine.

Another reason why current estrogen therapies have caused problems is that neither of the most common medications is well tolerated by humans. Premarin is actually equine (horse) estrogen, and humans don't have the metabolism to process it well. Provera is a synthetic chemical called medroxy progesterone, which the body doesn't metabolize in the same way that it does the natural hormones.

Strangely, there have been only limited tests of the effects of natural estrogens. Preliminary results from the most recent U.S. National Health and Nutrition Examination Survey indicate that natural estrogens offer most of the same benefits of estrogen replacement but without any demonstrable risk.

Somewhat less controversial are the findings that estrogen may be an effective antidepressant for depressed women. Scientists at the NIMH found that 80 percent of depressed women suffering with problems of irritability, sadness, and sleep disturbances showed improvement with hormone replacement therapy (HRT).

If You Are Cooling Deficient and Have PMS

A study by researchers at the University of Reading in England showed that a daily cocktail of 200 mg of magnesium and 50 mg of B-6 was modestly effective in reducing PMS-related anxiety and irritability.

Perhaps the best option is to ask your doctor about SSRIs. Over thirty clinical trials have demonstrated that these serotonin-enhancing drugs are effective in reducing the physical and emotional symptoms of PMS. If you're concerned about taking these drugs on a regular basis (some of the side effects are less than desirable), recent indications are that taking them during the luteal phase of your cycle is just as effective as taking them every day.

Naturally we recommend that you check with your gynecologist before starting any treatment, whether it's natural, hormonal, or prescription-based. Any of these may conflict with other medications you're currently taking.

Prescription Drugs

Drugs can act as either cooling agonists (meaning they enhance cooling effects) or antagonists (meaning they block them). Agonists include Zoloft and Paxil for depression, generalized anxiety, panic attacks, and PTSD, and Gabitril for seizures. Some work specifically on serotonin, others on GABA. Drugs that increase serotonin or GABA generally do so by blocking absorption by the body, which results in a net increase in cooling neurotransmitters in the cellular neighborhoods that need them most. Other drugs may work by blocking one or more of the warming neurotransmitters, particularly dopamine and glutamate.

Your physician and/or psychiatrist have access to a number of antidepressants and other pharmacological agents that can increase the production and release of serotonin and or GABA. As always, even though you may be 100 percent sure on your own that you have a

GABA or serotonin deficiency, don't start taking any of these drugs without consulting a trained medical professional. Just because a friend or relative may be taking one of the drugs we discuss below doesn't mean it will work for you. In addition, some of these drugs work in strange ways and you want to have your reactions to the drugs monitored by someone who knows what to look for.

Drugs That Increase Serotonin

SSRIs.   Selective serotonin reuptake inhibitors are widely used to treat depression, panic attacks, PTSD, OCD, and social phobias. The most common are Zoloft, Paxil, Prozac, Celexa, Effexor, and Lexapro. All of the SSRIs are similar in that they all increase serotonin levels in the brain. But they're different in a number of important ways, particularly when it comes to their specific uses and side effects. One important aspect of SSRIs is the effect they have— directly or indirectly—on dopamine. As serotonin increases, a possible unwanted consequence may be to reduce brain dopamine levels. Dopamine reduction is responsible for the common side effects of SSRIs, such as weight gain, decreased libido and/or sexual function, fatigue, and memory disturbances. Zoloft and Prozac are the least likely to lower dopamine levels, and there's some evidence that they actually raise them. This makes Zoloft and Prozac good choices in treating anhedonic depression that is marked by fatigue. Paxil increases norepinephrine, which makes it better suited to treat anxiety. In low doses, Effexor inhibits the uptake of serotonin, and in higher doses, it inhibits uptake of norepinephrine. Side effects of most SSRIs include dizziness, nausea, and some sexual problems. Celexa and Lexapro have no effects on dopamine one way or the other. Despite marketing materials that claim little or no weight gain or sexual side effects, our patients tell us otherwise. Overall, because of dopamine-depleting effects, many psychiatrists combine SSRIs with Wellbutrin or Provigil, two dopamine-enhancing drugs. Use SSRIs with caution if you have high blood pressure or kidney problems and never take them if you're taking an MAO inhibitor.

Ability *(aripipazole)*.   The first of a new class of drugs called *dopamine-serotonin stabilizers*. Abilify has the capacity to block either or both of these neurotransmitters. See page 271 for more.

The Downside to SSRIs

Although SSRIs appear to be beneficial in treating a wide variety of conditions, there can be some risks involved. A recent study published in the *Archives of Pediatric Adolescent Medicine* found a possible link between childhood treatment with SSRIs and a stunted growth spurt during puberty. Additional research is ongoing.

One of the most disturbing (albeit rather rare) possibilities when taking an SSRI is the loss of the ability to feel pleasure, a condition called *anhedonia.* The exact mechanism for this problem is not known, but researchers believe it is unrelated to the loss of the ability to achieve or the delay in reaching orgasm observed in both men and women taking SSRIs. The sexual side effects can be mitigated by augmenting the SSRI with a warming agent such as Wellbutrin, but there is no way to offset the problem of anhedonia. Fortunately this does not happen very often. And when it does, there are other cooling-enhancing options to try.

Serotonin syndrome (SS) is a condition that is caused by an excess of serotonin. It usually results from taking too much of a serotonin agonist (including the drug Ecstasy) or from combining SSRIs or L-tryptophan with MAO inhibitors (drugs that block production of *monoamine oxidase,* a chemical that breaks down dopamine in the brain) or St. John's wort. Symptoms may include:

- restlessness, irritability, or anxiety
- dizziness, confusion, or delirium
- nausea, vomiting, or diarrhea
- muscle rigidity, tremors, or loss of coordination
- irregular heart rate or shivering

If you are taking an SSRI or any other serotonin agonist and experience any of those, call your doctor immediately. About 80 percent of the time, serotonin syndrome symptoms disappear within a week after the offending drug or drug combination is stopped. But before taking yourself off any prescription drugs, make sure you talk to the doctor who prescribed them.

Drugs That Increase GABA and/or Block Glutamate

GABA plays a vital role in cognition, pain, sleep, and anxiety, but the hitch to increasing GABA is that it doesn't cross the blood-brain barrier. For that reason, taking ordinary GABA supplements is a complete waste of time and money—they may raise blood levels but they do nothing for brain levels. The solution is to take drugs that work like GABA but that trick the cells that form the blood-brain barrier into letting them through. That's exactly how drugs such as Valium, Xanax, and Ativan work. Rather than actually increasing GABA production, these drugs actually bind to the GABA receptors and produce the same effect.

Another approach to increasing GABA activity is to block its absorption in the same way that SSRIs inhibit the uptake of serotonin. Gabitril (tiagabine) is a member of a new class of drugs, the SGRIs (selective GABA reuptake inhibitors). Gabitril is frequently used to treat epilepsy, but many doctors are finding it useful in patients with anxiety, sleep problems, and chronic conditions.

Other drugs that influence GABA include the benzodiazepines, drugs that suppress overall brain activity and reduce anxiety. Side effects include sedation and memory problems. Others include Depakote, Neurontin, and Lamictal.

A number of glutamate-blocking antiseizure medications, particularly the ones mentioned in the previous paragraph, have proven beneficial to bipolar patients, as well as those with chronic pain conditions.

Lithium is another glutamate antagonist, which makes it a GABA agonist at the same time. It's a naturally occurring substance that exists in trace amounts in the body as well as in plants and minerals. It's been used to treat manic patients since the mid 1970s. Lithium is sometimes used in conjunction with other, more traditional antidepressants for bipolar disease. Unfortunately, it's effective in only about half of patients. One of the problems is that the dosage depends on the weight of the patient and must therefore be monitored constantly and carefully to minimize risk of kidney or thyroid problems. In conjunction with divalproex sodium, lithium was shown to be extremely effective in treating pathological gambling, according to a recent study published in the *Journal of Clinical Psychiatry*. Side effects of lithium include gastrointestinal symptoms, weight gain, acne, tremors, sedation, and loss of coordination. Lithium shouldn't be taken with Advil or Motrin, diuretics, and some antibiotics, such as erythromycin, because all of these raise lithium levels, which can throw off the dose.

A new device called a *vagal nerve stimulator* has recently been approved for epilepsy and also for people with depression. Implanted in the neck, the device works kind of like a pacemaker, electronically stimulating the nerve. Although researchers aren't quite sure how or why it works, the theory is that increasing the parasympathetic nervous system reduces the release of glutamate in the brain, which is one of the major causes of seizures. The stimulator has been especially successful for patients who either can't tolerate or don't respond to the traditional antiseizure medications (Depakote, Neurontin, etc.).

EEG Biofeedback (Neurofeedback)

Neurofeedback is a technique designed to teach you how to regulate your own brain waves. We're including it in this section because it's a process that you have to be taught, but you generally can't get in to see a biofeedback professional without a physician referral. EEG measures and quantifies electrical brain wave activity in various parts of the brain.

Biofeedback techniques may take a while to master—as many as fifty one-hour sessions—but results can be dramatic and permanent.

Now that you've reached the end of this 28-day plan to boost your cooling neurotransmitters, you're feeling less depressed, less tense, emotionally stable, and more in control of your weight. Actually, this isn't really the end, it's the beginning. In order to retain your current level of balance—or to fine-tune it even further—you'll have to make this plan a daily habit. Don't feel overwhelmed: you don't have to be 100 percent perfect every second of every day. If you miss a workout or have an extra piece of chocolate cake once in a while, you'll be okay. But if you let things go too far, the symptoms that led you to buy this book in the first place will come back. Because gradual changes sometimes go unnoticed, we suggest that you retake the quiz in chapter 2 every few months or so, and that you get back on the plan immediately before you start feeling bad again.

CHAPTER 8

Getting Back in Balance

Overcoming Your Dual
Neurotransmitter Deficit

Prolonged stress can deplete the brain's ability to produce adequate amounts of warming and cooling neurotransmitters. This may have left you with a number of seemingly contradictory complaints, such as low energy and restlessness, depression and anxiousness, chronic fatigue and chronic pain, cravings for cigarettes, caffeine, alcohol, or tranquilizers, and a combination of internally and externally directed anger.

To expand on a point we introduced in chapter 5, combined deficits of warming and cooling NTs are usually brought on by prolonged psychological and/or physical stress, which unleash several chemical reactions that cause actual physical damage to the brain. These chemical reactions include the release of excess cortisol and glutamate, increased production of free radicals, and a breakdown of lipid or fat membranes that surround brain cells. They also cause an overproduction of *heat shock proteins.* In general, heat shock proteins are a good thing; they act as the brain's janitors, cleaning up and removing cellular debris that could otherwise clutter up your brain. But when heat shock protein levels get too high—which happens during periods of high stress—they remove healthy cellular material as well.

Treating a dual deficiency is no more complicated than treating a single deficiency. Our simple rule is this: *If you're deficient in both warming and cooling NTs, treat the cooling deficit first.* Why? Think of it this way: a cooling deficiency is, almost by definition, a warming excess. And if you increase warming NTs, you're literally adding fuel to the fire. Stimulating someone who's already experiencing anxiety, nervousness, panic, withdrawal, or fear will aggravate those cooling-deficient symptoms, making it impossible for the patient to tolerate the treatment.

Imagine trying to train a wild animal. The first step is to get the animal to trust you. If you can't do that, you'll never be able to overcome the animal's fear and aggression. The same goes for dual deficiencies. By correcting the cooling side of the deficiency first, we're effectively building trust and feelings of safety in your brain and nervous system. Without that solid foundation of trust and safety, any attempts to address the warming deficiency will fail.

In order to better understand—and treat—your dual deficiency, we want you to follow the entire 28-day cooling deficiency program in chapter 7:

- perspective, including banishing negative thinking
- sleep, making sure you get at least seven and a half hours a night
- exercise, including aerobics and gentle stretching
- lifestyle, focusing on relaxation and meditation
- diet

However, we've made two important changes that will offset the destructive biochemical impact of your dual deficiency and protect your brain.

Perspective

In addition to the perspective and affirmations you do as part of the cooling program, remember that moderation is the key to your recovery. What does moderation mean? Mostly it means being flexible. Take this program, for example. If you inadvertently skip your affirmation one day or miss a day of exercise, let it go. Just make an extra effort to do all the activities the next day. If you're too busy to exercise one day, park at the far end of the parking lot and walk briskly to wherever you're going. Or consider taking the stairs instead of the elevator. If you can't do the full amount of meditation, do as much as you can.

Flexibility is important in the rest of your life too. If you're faced with a choice or an opportunity, take the middle road whenever possible and avoid extremes. Set realistic goals. Saying you're going to quit smoking or lose twenty-five pounds by the end of the year may be setting yourself up for disappointment. Instead, break it down into more manageable increments, such as cutting down your smoking by a pack a week or losing half a pound a week. That will enable you to celebrate many small successes along the way.

And finally, take care of one thing at a time. As we've said, dual deficiencies are most often caused by extended or severe stress. Trying to deal with five or six stressors at the same time will only make you feel worse. Instead, resolve one as much as you can before moving on to the next one.

Supplements

The second important change from the single-deficit cooling plan to the cooling plan that's part of a dual-deficit program is that this plan includes different nutritional, herbal, and amino acid supplements. People with dual deficits are in a precarious state of neurotransmitter balance. Making changes in perspective, sleep, exercise, lifestyle, and diet raises cooling NTs gently so as to not upset that balance or aggravate the patient's symptoms. But when it comes to chemical means (including nutritional, herbal, and amino acid supplements), the changes can be too sudden and can cause *paradox,* meaning that the supplements used to treat one deficit could make the other deficit even worse.

For that reason, the supplements that we use to treat patients with dual deficiencies generally increase both warming and cooling NTs at the same time. These include fatty acids and herbs.

Fatty Acids

- *Phosphatidylserine (PS).* A fatty acid compound that forms part of the structural layer of biological membranes in brain cells. PS plays a role in the complicated process of *signal transduction,* supporting the dynamic interaction between neurotransmitters and their receptors in the brain, conveying NT messages into the interior of the cell. An over-the-counter PS compound is frequently used as an anti-stress supplement because of its ability to decrease cortisol and raise brain serotonin.

- EPA and DHA.   The most important of the essential fatty acids. They include omega-3 and typically come in softgels that provide 300 mg of EPA and 200 mg of DHA.

Herbs

- *Withania* (also called *Ashwaganda*).   An anti-inflammatory herb used in Ayurvedic medicine to promote physical and mental health. In a variety of studies, withania has reduced cortisol levels in the blood, improved sleep, elevated and stabilized mood, and calmed frazzled nerves. Besides increasing serotonin and dopamine, this remarkable herb activates certain acetylcholine receptors, which may explain withania's positive effects on clarity of thinking and memory. One very important warning about Ayurvedic herbs: many of the ones imported directly from India are contaminated with heavy metals. Several American companies also produce these herbs, and they're much safer. Don't buy any Indian herbs from a company that doesn't guarantee that the product is pure and heavy-metal free. Your best bet is to ask the pharmacist at a major drug-store or nutritional supplement chain to recommend a reliable, quality-assured brand.
- *Reishi mushroom extract.*   Extract of the mushroom *Ganoderma lucidum.* For about 2,000 years it's been used to treat a variety of ailments, including hepatitis and other liver conditions. Reishi extract is known to reduce blood pressure, decrease bad cholesterol levels, increase white blood cells, and facilitate the transport of nutrients and oxygen through the body. Insomniacs have used it to relax muscles and increase sleeping time, and many in Asia use it to enhance their immune system or as a cancer treatment.

The Newest Weapon in the Battle against Free Radicals

We know that free radicals work with excessive levels of glutamate to damage the neurons that produce both dopamine and serotonin. Fortunately, our brain comes equipped with a built-in defense mechanism: a natural antioxidant called *superoxide dismutase,* or SOD. Research has shown that SOD levels gradually decrease as we age. But they drop off precipitously during and after severe or chronic stress or neurodegenerative conditions such as Alzheimer's, Parkinson's, and chronic fatigue syndrome.

SOD cannot be taken orally because it's broken down by our digestive enzymes and it never makes it to where it's supposed to go. But recently a team of French scientists discovered how to produce SOD from cantaloupe and other melons, and they combined it with a wheat protein called *gliadin* to produce the first orally active SOD compound that doesn't lose its antioxidant properties in our stomach. This gliadin-SOD mixture is called *GliSODin,* and it's an important ingredient in two novel products called Resurgex and Prosurgex, both manufactured by Millennium Biotechnologies, Inc. In preliminary studies, people taking GliSODin reported reduced fatigue and generally improved well-being.

For the first fourteen days of the program, take the following supplements:

- 200 mg *phosphatidylserine* (PS), twice a day, with food
- 900 mg EPA per day, with food
- 600 mg DHA per day, with food
- 500 mg withania per day. Start off at the low end and increase the dosage as necessary.
- 100 mg reishi mushroom extract per day
- 500 mg GliSODin per day. *Warning: If you have a gliadin sensitivity or a wheat allergy, do not take GliSODin.* If you're not absolutely sure, check with your doctor before trying this antioxidant.

On days fifteen through twenty-eight, continue taking the same amount of PS, EPA, DHA, and GliSODin every day, but make the following changes:

- Increase withania to 1,000 mg per day
- Increase reishi mushroom extract to 300 mg per day
- Take 100 mg of 5-HTP one hour after supper

In addition, take the following every morning with breakfast:

- 800 mcg folate
- 100 mg B-6
- 500 mg inositol
- 400 mg magnesium

Working with Your Doctor to Get Back in Balance

Although most dual neurotransmitter deficiencies can be treated without medical intervention, some people may need some extra help in the form of hormones and prescription drugs that can (or should) be prescribed only by a trained medical professional. Again, none of the drugs or compounds in this section should be taken in any quantity except under the direction of your doctor.

Hormones

DHEA

DHEA is a perfectly safe hormone found in the adrenal glands as well as in the *glial cells* that make up the blood-brain barrier. DHEA acts on both warming and cooling neurotransmitters and produces a number of effects. It raises brain levels of both norepinephrine and serotonin, enhances the neurons' excitability, and improves their plasticity (their ability to grow and adapt in response to experience). It is also involved in regulating the balance between glutamate and GABA, which is critical in memory formation and retention.

DHEA also helps your metabolism by breaking down fat in the body and making it available for conversion into usable energy. It modulates immune cell activities, offsets the action of the stress hormone cortisol, and in animal studies is very effective in lowering the body temperature. DHEA is also commonly prescribed by psychiatrists for treatment of postmenopausal depression. Although DHEA is available over the counter, it's still a hormone and should be treated as such. That means that you should never take it unless you're under medical supervision.

Thyroid

Patients with depression, anxiety, or mixed anxiety-depressive disorder are at greater risk of having thyroid problems—either underactive (hypothyroidism) or overactive (hyperthyroidism). Approximately 10 to 15 percent of depressed patients have thyroid deficiency, and most patients with thyroid deficiency have signs of depression. Some people speculate that psychiatric and thyroid diseases share a common biological origin. Thyroid therapy has been effective in reducing depressive and anxiety symptoms.

Prescription Drugs

Medical Cocktails

Dealing with dual deficiencies sometimes requires targeting both warming and cooling neurotransmitters at the same time. Many psychiatrists give their depressed patients a combination of Wellbutrin (a dopamine-increasing antidepressant) and Zoloft (a serotonin-increasing antidepressant) that they informally call Well-oft. This combination allows us to address dual deficiencies of dopamine and serotonin in a unique way. Wellbutrin by itself can be too stimulating for some patients, causing insomnia and undesired weight loss. Zoloft takes the edge off the Wellbutrin by increasing levels of calming, cooling neurotransmitters. On the other hand, Zoloft by itself often causes extreme fatigue and some very undesirable sexual side effects, including reduced libido and inability to reach orgasm. Stimulating warming NTs with Wellbutrin often relieves both the fatigue and the sexual problems.

Provigil (another dopamine-enhancing drug) used in place of Wellbutrin has been very effective in treating patients with depression and extreme fatigue or with severe cognitive deficits related to the depression.

Effexor

Effexor stimulates warming and cooling NTs in one pill. In this case, norepinephrine is the warming NT and serotonin the cooling. Effexor is also sometimes combined with Wellbutrin, enabling patients to increase three neurotransmitters at the same time: serotonin, norepinephrine, and dopamine.

Abilify

An amazing new class of drugs called *dopamine-serotonin stabilizers* has recently been developed. The first one to get FDA approval is *aripipazole,* sold as Abilify. Unlike drugs that block either serotonin or dopamine, Abilify has the remarkable capacity to do either or both. It acts like a thermostat, decreasing the synthesis of serotonin and dopamine in the brain when there's too much there, and increasing it if brain levels are too low. Abilify is approved for schizophrenia and psychosis but also may be effective in broader clinical applications, such as ADD, autism, OCD, bipolar disease, and Tourette's.

Lamictal

An antiseizure drug that increases serotonin and decreases glutamate, thereby helping to restore the GABA/glutamate balance. It is currently being used by psychiatrists to treat bipolar disease and has a distinct advantage over lithium, which prevents mania but doesn't do anything for the depressive symptoms. Lamictal does both. Lamictal may soon be available as an antidepressant. *Cautions:* Fewer than 1 percent of patients taking Lamictal develop a life-threatening rash.

Following the Cooling Program with the modified perspective and supplements for twenty-eight days will help you overcome your cooling-deficit symptoms and give you the strength and security you need to start working on your warming deficiency. However, if you have a more serious condition, such as bipolar disease, depression that isn't responding to treatment, autism, or ADHD and OCD combined, we strongly suggest that you talk to your physician about the prescription drugs that address both deficiencies simultaneously.

By the time you've finished this modified Cooling Program, there's a very good chance that your warming neurotransmitter levels will have improved as well. As counterintuitive as that sounds, it's true. When your warming neurotransmitter systems begin to feel safe and secure again, they may resume NT production on their own. Once you're done with the cooling program, go back and take the test in chapter 2 again. If you're still warming deficient, go ahead and do the 28-day Warming Program.

Because you're susceptible to deficiencies of both warming and cooling neurotransmitters, it's essential that you pay close attention to your symptoms and maintain a healthy lifestyle that will enable you to keep your levels of both NTs high and balanced. Doing so will give you control over your mental and physical health and will relegate the lack of mental sharpness, low energy, depression, anxiousness, anger, cravings, pain, and other symptoms to your past.

Conclusion

Congratulations on having finished a book that has more potential to change your life for the better than anything else you've ever read. Actually, you should congratulate *yourself*—you're the one who did it!

Learning about neurotransmitters and how they make you the person you are gives you tremendous power. You now possess the knowledge and insight to recognize what's going on when you don't feel as well as you'd like and the tools that will help you take quick and decisive steps to restore your unique balance.

But knowledge and tools are useless unless you put them to use. So we urge you to make them part of your life. Not just today or once in a while, but every single day for the rest of your life. If you do, the benefits to you, as well as your family and friends, will be fantastic.

When your warming and cooling neurotransmitters are properly balanced, you'll feel more energetic, alert, focused, joyful, safe, and calm. And that's just the beginning.

Additional benefits include:

- a more consistent energy level
- freedom from food, alcohol, sugar, caffeine, or drug cravings
- control over your weight and a lower percentage of body fat

- reduction of physical symptoms such as chronic pain or swelling, diminished sex drive, frequent colds or flu, migraines, and PMS and other menstrual disorders
- emotional stability
- greater satisfaction and contentment with life
- decreased hostility, panic, and anxiety
- improved sleep
- increased mental clarity, concentration, and decision-making ability
- better memory
- improved mood and emotional stability
- elimination of depression
- improved friendships and other relationships

We sincerely wish you the very best of luck on your path toward uncovering a healthier happier self.

RECOMMENDED READING

If you're interested in exploring in greater detail how warming and cooling neurotransmitters influence our lives and the links between mind and body, you might want to take a look at some or all of the following titles.

Austin, James. *Zen and the Brain: Toward an Understanding of Meditation and Consciousness.* MIT Press, 1999.

Damasio, Antonio. *The Feeling of What Happens: Body and Emotion in the Making of Consciousness.* Harvest Books, 2000.

Gleick, James. *Chaos: Making a New Science.* Penguin USA, 1998.

Kaptchuk, Ted. *The Web That Has No Weaver: Understanding Chinese Medicine.* McGraw-Hill/Contemporary Books, 2000.

Kramer, Peter. *Listening to Prozac.* Penguin, 1997.

Miller, Marlane. *Brainstyles: Change Your Life without Changing Who You Are.* Simon & Schuster, 1997.

Norden, Michael. *Beyond Prozac: Antidotes for Modern Times.* HarperCollins, 1996.

Pert, Candace. *Molecules of Emotions: The Science Behind Mind-Body Medicine.* Simon & Schuster, 1999.

Peterson, Jordan. *Maps of Meaning: The Architecture of Belief.* Routledge, 1999.

Ramachandran, V. S. *Phantoms in the Brain: Probing the Mysteries of the Human Mind.* Quill, 1999.

Siever, Larry. *The New View of Self: How Genes and Neurotransmitters Shape Your Mind, Your Personality, and Your Mental Health.* Diane Publishing Co, 1997.

If you're a researcher, a scientist, a physician, or especially interested in a deeper, more technical discussion, you may enjoy the following titles.

Cooper, Jack, et al. *The Biochemical Basis of Neuropharmacology.* Oxford University Press, 2002.

Davidson, Richard J., (editor), Kenneth Hugdahl (editor), *Brain Asymmetry.* MIT Press, 1996.

Furman, Mark and Fred Gallo. *Neurophysics of Human Behavior: Explorations at the Interface of the Brain, Mind, Behavior, and Information.* CRC Press, 2000.

Grilly, David. *Drugs and Human Behavior.* Allyn & Bacon, 2001.

Robertson, David, (editor) et al, *Primmer on the Automatic Nervous System.* Academic Press, 1996.

Stahl, Stephen M. and Nancy Muntner, *Essential Psychopharmacology of Antipsychotics and Mood Stabilizers.* Cambridge University Press, 2002.

Stahl, Stephen M. and Nancy Muntner, *Essential Psychopharmacology: Neuroscientific Basis and Practical Applications.* Cambridge University Press, 2000.

Webster, Roy, (editor), *Neurotransmitters, Drugs, and Brain Function.* John Wiley & Sons, 2001.

Wolfram, Stephen. *A New Kind of Science.* Wolfram Media, 2002.

Appendix

Purchasing Supplements

You can purchase the supplements we recommend in our 28-day programs at most health food stores as well as on the Internet. However, because of the potential problems with quality assurance and the purity of ingredients, we strongly recommend that you ask your retailer for a guarantee that the product you are buying is of the highest quality and reliability.

For your convenience, you can also purchase these supplements—quality and reliability assured—through our Web site at www.advancedbrainchemistry.com or by calling 1-800-460-1959. We also invite you to regularly visit the site for the latest information on new developments in the field of neuroscience and new products that we feel may help you keep your brain and your life in balance.

INDEX